PREVENTING MEDICATION ERRORS AT HOME

PREVENTING MEDICATION ERRORS AT HOME

SIMON HAROUTOUNIAN

OXFORD
UNIVERSITY PRESS

OXFORD
UNIVERSITY PRESS

Oxford University Press is a department of the University of Oxford. It furthers
the University's objective of excellence in research, scholarship, and education
by publishing worldwide. Oxford is a registered trade mark of Oxford University
Press in the UK and certain other countries.

Published in the United States of America by Oxford University Press
198 Madison Avenue, New York, NY 10016, United States of America.

Library of Congress Cataloging-in-Publication Data
Names: Haroutounian, Simon, author.
Title: Preventing medication errors at home / Simon Haroutounian.
Description: New York, NY : Oxford University Press, [2019]
Identifiers: LCCN 2019009451| ISBN 9780190674984 (hardback) |
ISBN 9780190674991 (updf) | ISBN 9780190675004 (epub)
Subjects: LCSH: Drugs—Popular works. | Medication errors—Prevention.
Classification: LCC RS91 .H37 2019 | DDC 615.1-dc23
LC record available at https://lccn.loc.gov/2019009451

9 8 7 6 5 4 3 2 1

Printed by Sheridan Books, Inc., United States of America

to Ruben and Tori

—You can do anything you set your mind to. Take the risk of failing, keep trying, and do not give up.

to Dina,

—Thank you for teaching me kindness, fairness, compassion, and friendship. You are the love of my life.

CONTENTS

PART II
MEDICATION THERAPY TIPS IN COMMON DISEASE STATES

ACKNOWLEDGMENTS

There are several people without whom this book would never have happened.

When I first thought about writing a comprehensive book about drugs for the general readership, I had concerns about how it would be perceived, and somewhat doubted my own ability to take on such a heavy lift. I am indebted to my friend, Ariel Averbuch, for encouraging me to get out of my comfort zone and become more time-efficient to make meaningful things like this happen. Thank you for believing in me and pushing me at times of self-doubt.

I will be forever thankful to my mentor and dear friend, Arthur G. Lipman, for introducing me to the field of pain management, where I found my clinical and research passion. Thank you for more than 10 years of endless wisdom, support, and optimism. Rest in peace, Art, I miss you every day.

I am thankful to Craig Panner, editor at Oxford University Press, for providing a fresh perspective, a keen editorial eye, and unbelievable patience with (what seemed to be an endless process of) revisions and rewriting to make the book more comprehensible to the general audience.

ACKNOWLEDGMENTS

I have been truly fortunate to have outstanding teachers and mentors who have taught me, and have encouraged me to think, about safe and effective use of medications. I cannot list all of these individuals and apologize for omitting some. Amnon Hoffman, Elyad Davidson, Evan Kharasch, Maya Lodzki, and Oren Shavit—I am eternally grateful.

PART I

EVERYTHING YOU NEED
TO KNOW ABOUT DRUGS

[1]

PRESCRIPTION MEDICATIONS

Friend or Foe?

"My drugs are killing me." This is a phrase I have heard many times from patients. "This drug causes heartburn, the other makes me drowsy, these two cause constipation." These statements from people who use prescription medications raise legitimate but tough questions: Are these drugs doing us any good? Are they really necessary?

One thing is certain: as a society, we consume quite a lot of medications these days. Fifty percent of all people in the United States and 80% of adults older than 50 years use at least one prescription drug. About 40% of people older than 60 years use five or more prescription drugs on a monthly basis, and it is not uncommon for adults older than 60 years to use 10 to 15 daily prescription medications. But how much do we benefit from these drugs, and does their benefit surpass the potential risks?

So let's first take a brief tour through the history of medication use and through some facts so that you can shape your own opinion on the matter. My hope is that the current chapter and the book as a whole will improve your factual knowledge base and assist you in recognizing the true benefits and risks associated with drug treatment.

A LITTLE BIT OF HISTORY ON THE USE OF REMEDIES

The practice of medicine, or healing, dates back to approximately the 30th century BCE: that's at least 4500 years of providing remedies to people to ease their pain and suffering. Early methods for treating ailments used herbs, plants, and animal byproducts, often as a part of religious or spiritual ceremonies. This knowledge of the healing properties of natural products had been acquired through trial and error and was typically passed on verbally and in the form of treatment rituals from generation to generation of healers in the various ancient societies. The first *written* evidence of organized (or *systematic*—if you will) treatment of diseases dates back 3500 years to ancient Egyptian documents such as the Edwin Smith Papyrus (approx. 1600 BCE) and the Ebers Papyrus (approx. 1500 BCE), which contain quite detailed descriptions of remedies to treat physical and mental illnesses. Babylonian, Chinese, and Indian texts from approximately the 12th to 8th centuries BCE contain additional details on human physiology and pathology and describe treatment approaches. Some of these ancient texts describe treatments that are still relevant today, perhaps in somewhat modified forms, and include garlic, honey, cannabis plants, opium poppy extract, castor bean oil, and many other herbal remedies. It was not until the 4th century BCE, however, that the modern approach to medicine began to form, based on Hippocrates' systematic work on disease categorization (e.g., acute, chronic, epidemic), diagnosis, prognosis, and treatment. The understanding of how the human body works and how diseases occur continued to develop through outstanding efforts of physicians, scientists, and philosophers such as Galen (2nd century), Paracelsus and Vesalius (both 16th century), and many others.

EMERGENCE OF THE "DRUG" CONCEPT

It was only beginning in the mid-19th century that the modern principles of *pharmacology* [from Greek φάρμακον (drug, poison); and -λογία (the study of)], or the systematic study of the activity of substances on a body, were developed. In the late 19th century, John Newport Langley, a British physiologist, and Paul Ehrlich, a Nobel Prize–winning German immunologist, developed—somewhat independently—the basis for "drug receptor theory." Without knowing how exactly various compounds exert their action in the body, Langley discussed the existence of "receptive substance" in the tissues, and Ehrlich suggested his concept of *corpora non agunt nisi fixata*—"compounds only work when they are bound"—based on his numerous experiments with agents to kill microbial pathogens. What became known as *drug receptor theory* provided the basis for the modern drug development approach, the process that identifies a target involved in the disease process (i.e., the **receptor**) and discovers a **drug** compound that binds and either activates or inactivates this receptor target.

This target to which the drug needs to bind can be a virus that infects the lungs, an immune cell, or a certain protein in the body that is responsible for a disease process—for example, one that causes inflammation. The relevant drugs, in each such scenario, will have different activities: in the first case, the drug will exert *antiviral* activity; in the second case, it may be useful for treating *allergies*; and the third drug may be useful for *arthritis*. Regardless of what the receptor target is, we want the drug–receptor interaction to follow a **key–lock principle**, whereby the drug is the key and the receptor is the lock. The goal is that each drug only binds to and acts on its intended receptor target but spares other receptors, in the same way that we want our house key to open only our door. In the previous examples, it would be undesirable if the antiviral drug affected our joints, or if the arthritis medication had a negative effect on our immune cells.

EMERGENCE OF SINGLE DRUGS AS A REPLACEMENT FOR PLANT EXTRACTS

To follow the key–lock principle, modern drugs typically contain a single *active compound*—or, in other words, a measured amount of identical molecules. This is in contrast to the traditional plant extracts, which may sometimes contain dozens or hundreds of various compounds in addition to the active molecule we are interested in. While the compounds that don't occur in nature need to be synthesized in the laboratory, the naturally occurring compounds can be either synthesized or extracted from plants using chemical methods. To illustrate this: squeezing an orange will give you juice that contains vitamin C and many other compounds, such as those that give orange its color, odor, and taste. You can use the squeezed orange juice as a source of vitamin C, but it will contain other compounds that you may or may not want to consume. If you are only interested in the effect of vitamin C, you can get a vitamin C product in which all vitamin C molecules were extracted from fruit, or another product in which all vitamin C molecules were synthesized in a laboratory (and these would be the same molecules of vitamin C).

The first identified active compound used as a drug was *morphine*, isolated around 1805 from an opium poppy by Friedrich Sertürner—a pharmacist's apprentice in Paderborn (now central Germany). Sertürner described his process of isolating crystals of some unknown compound from the poppy, and he found that the compound induced sleep in rats and dogs (hence the drug was named after Morpheus, the ancient Greek god of dreams). One day Sertürner had a terrible toothache, and the pain prevented him from falling asleep. He swallowed a small amount of the compound and discovered not only that he fell asleep but also that the medicine provided incredible pain relief. And today, more than 200 years later, morphine is still one of the most widely used and powerful analgesics available.

The first *synthetic* drug (chemically produced in a laboratory, rather than extracted from a plant as morphine was) was *chloral hydrate*, which was first synthesized in 1832 by the German chemist Justus von Liebig. Later, in 1869, another German scientist, Oscar Liebreich, discovered that chloral hydrate has sedative properties. Following this discovery, chloral hydrate was in use for many years as a sedative to induce sleep and relieve anxiety during unpleasant procedures, particularly in children.

Although the activity of many of the early drugs was discovered by accident, just as in the examples with morphine and chloral hydrate, perhaps the first example of purposeful, or *rational,* drug development is presented by the synthesis of *acetylsalicylic acid*, known (and referred to in this book) as **aspirin**. The bark of the willow tree (genus *Salix*) contains *salicylic acid* and had been used for treating pain and inflammation for thousands of years. Willow, in fact, is mentioned as early as in the Ebers Papyrus (around 1500 BCE) and in Hippocrates' works (around 300 BCE). But salicylic acid was irritating to the stomach when taken by mouth. In 1897, Felix Hoffmann, a chemist working for the German pharmaceutical company Bayer, found that a minor chemical modification of salicylic acid to create *acetylsalicylic acid* reduced the stomach-irritating properties of the plant compound, while maintaining its therapeutic effect. And this is how aspirin—the first blockbuster drug—was introduced, and the era of large-scale drug manufacturing began.

DO DRUGS REALLY HELP?

In the 20th to 10th centuries BCE, the life expectancy was approximately 26 years. Thousands of years later, the average life expectancy worldwide in the 1950s was still less than 50 years, but it has dramatically increased throughout the past half-century to more than 70 years, with some countries currently reaching average life expectancy greater than 80 years. There are many potential factors that could have influenced this shift: decreased rates of infant mortality and fewer epidemics, plagues, wars, and accidents affecting younger people. However, even if we account for all these factors, our current *improved ability to treat chronic diseases* has played an extraordinary role in extending longevity.

Once considered deadly, many diseases, such as diabetes, infections, and certain types of cancer, can now be well controlled. This often allows people to gain near-normal quality of life despite having a serious underlying condition. As a result, more than 100 million people in the United States live with at least one chronic (long-term) disease, such as high blood pressure, diabetes, heart disease, or asthma. As populations age, however, the burden of age-related chronic conditions (especially those such as Alzheimer's disease and arthritis) is expected to steadily increase, and we face new challenges that require further research and novel solutions.

In the 1960s, more than 600 of every 100,000 people in the United States died of *heart disease* every year. Today, this rate has fallen by about 70%, to less than 200 of 100,000 people. The mortality rates from heart disease in most European countries have been following a similar trend. The overall picture of mortality following *stroke* is not much different either: stroke mortality rates per 100,000 population have fallen in the past 40 years in the United States, Australia, United Kingdom, and other European countries from about 150 to less than 50—again, about a 70% reduction in mortality. Is it all attributable to medications? Not necessarily. Diet, smoking cessation, better physical activity, and improved surgical and in-hospital interventions play an important role. But again, when these factors have been accounted for in hundreds of clinical trials, the beneficial effects of many drugs on preventing death, reducing hospitalizations, and improving quality of life are **undeniable**. To name just a few examples:

- Use of drugs for tighter control of blood pressure can reduce death rates by up to 40 to 50% over a few years.
- Use of *statin* drugs (see Chapter 12) in high-risk patients with high cholesterol levels can reduce the chance of heart attacks or death due to heart disease by 30 to 50%.
- HIV medications, when taken in appropriate combination "cocktails," can almost eliminate AIDS symptoms and allow close to normal quality of life in many patients.
- Many infectious diseases that used to be deadly are easily controlled today by antibiotics.
- Inhaled corticosteroids (see Chapter 15), when taken regularly as prescribed, can reduce the chance of hospitalization due to asthma attacks by 80%.

And this factual list goes on and on, suggesting that drugs can truly be our friends, especially for managing chronic diseases. So do drugs really help? I think the answer is "certainly yes." Are all drugs safe and beneficial? The answer is "certainly not!"

WHEN DRUGS ARE NOT USED APPROPRIATELY

Millions of people have been harmed by drugs: excessive bleeding caused by unmonitored use of blood thinners such as aspirin and warfarin, birth abnormalities in children whose mothers were exposed to *teratogenic*[1] drugs such as diethylstilbestrol and isotretinoin, serious liver damage caused by antiepileptic drugs such as valproate and phenytoin, deaths from (intentional or unintentional) overdose of opioid analgesics—you name it. But as in many areas in our lives—it's all a matter of **risk-to-benefit ratio**.

You would not ban people from driving cars or using public transportation despite the risk for motor vehicle collisions (40,000 deaths a year in the United States alone), and you would not ban women from giving birth despite 24,000 annual fetal deaths in the United States. I hope you agree with me that the solution would be to improve safety and do the maximum to protect the individuals at risk in both these categories. By illustrating the potential risks and dangers in using medications and by providing the insight to make safe and intelligent decisions about your treatment, this book can help prevent medication errors at home.

For the general question of "to use or not to use medications at all"—the balance **by far** tips to the side of "to use." On the other hand, we are far from using the available medications safely—and there still are substantial risks associated with drug use. The 1 million drug-related hospital admissions and 40,000 to 80,000 prescription drug–related deaths every year in the United States are terrifying statistics that certainly support the latter point that the safe use of medications still requires substantial education.

So where do we go from here? There are ongoing studies investigating the causes of drug-associated damage, trying to understand how and in whom this damage occurs. As the scientific knowledge base grows, patients should try to educate themselves with information from reliable sources in order to implement that knowledge in a way that is relevant to the health of themselves and their loved ones.

---

1. *Teratogenic* substances are those that increase the risk for birth abnormalities when pregnant women are exposed to them.

Most undesired drug effects that could be prevented by the healthcare team happen at **prescribing** and **monitoring** stages. Several studies have shown that the most common drug error that leads to serious consequences, such as hospitalization, is the *wrong drug* (or *inappropriate drug*) type of error (in 40 to 75% of patients), especially in older adults. What this type of error means is that the prescribed drug was not appropriate for treating the persons' particular condition, or it should not have been prescribed to that individual because of factors such as their age, weight, other medications, or other existing conditions. Lack of appropriate monitoring of drugs such as blood thinners, diabetes drugs, and diuretics (colloquially called *water pills*) is another major cause of drug-associated hospitalizations.

In 1999, the Institute of Medicine described the concerning state of medical errors on a large scale in "To Err Is Human." This report suggested that about 50% of the drug-associated errors were preventable, and it proposed a roadmap for building a safer hospital system. That is certainly easier said than done. We could wait (who knows for how many years) until such a safe hospital system is in place. But a safer hospital system is not going to solve the main problem: most drug-related errors occur at home, where most people take their medications, outside the hospital setting. Even if an excellent physician accurately made your diagnosis and prescribed the most appropriate medication for your condition, and the pharmacist correctly dispensed it, that would still not ensure your safety. If you take your medication in an improper manner, or use another drug that counteracts the prescribed medicine (or increases its toxicity) without first consulting your doctor or pharmacist, no healthcare system in the world can keep you safe. In contrast, educating yourself about the potential dangers of drugs and the ways to ensure better treatment outcomes for your conditions can serve you well in both the short term and the long run.

An interesting and careful study conducted by Friedman and colleagues in 2007 looked at causes of medication errors in a group of high-risk patients (who received kidney, liver, or pancreas transplants). Among 93 patients who participated in the study, 143 medication errors were identified—which is **more than one error for every patient**. On average, each patient was treated with 11 drugs, and almost 20% of the participants in this observational study (17 out of 93) had been hospitalized because of drug side effects during the first year after their transplant surgery. Although a certain proportion of the overall errors were healthcare team errors, nearly 70% of the errors were patient errors. This confirms my previous suggestion that regardless of safety improvements to the healthcare system, it is only when the patients are sufficiently educated and responsible for their own drugs that the majority of drug-associated damage can be prevented.

And the good news is that the medical literature shows that between 50 and 70% of drug-related complications and deaths are indeed *preventable*. On a population level, we have not figured out what is the best way to educate patients to prevent these errors, but my contribution, through the information in this book, is to share the current knowledge and my experience to help you guide your drug treatment toward achieving your therapy goals in a safer manner, and hence to help you live a longer and healthier life.

Take-Home Message

Many medications have the proven benefits of saving and prolonging lives, increasing life quality, and alleviating pain and suffering. However, they will do so safely only when properly prescribed, taken, and monitored. There are potential risks associated with drug treatments, sometimes as serious as hospitalization or death. Learning about your medical conditions and carefully educating yourself about the risks and benefits of your drugs can help you prevent unnecessary complications and achieve a life of better quality and longer duration.

[2]

WHY DO I NEED
TO UNDERSTAND MY
DRUGS BETTER?

In this chapter, I will discuss two fundamental concepts that provide the basis for physician-patient communication about medications. In virtually any decision-making process, a clear understanding of risks and benefits promotes a more responsible course of action and helps achieve better results. Many successful smoking cessation programs, as well as exercise and diet programs, are based on the idea that the better informed you are, the better the success rates will be. Look at the success of breast and cervical cancer screening programs: they save tens of thousands lives every year. Even in young children, clearly outlining risks and benefits is shown to promote positive behavior such as regular brushing of teeth and consumption of vegetables. And the more in-depth the educational process, the better the results.

In all the previous examples, a **one-way** communication of benefits and risks almost NEVER works, especially in the long run. After the initial educational process, a response is always required on behalf of the "learner." This response then needs to be followed by a feedback process to reinforce further correct action. It's no different with medications, only that the terms benefit and risk are replaced by effectiveness and safety. A good understanding of what these terms mean in relation to *your drugs* is going to be critical for obtaining good health.

ASSESSING DRUG EFFECTIVENESS AND SAFETY

Allow me to begin from the very basics. I mentioned the *drug receptor theory* in Chapter 1, and the fact that it guides the researchers and the clinicians to understand how drugs work. Usually, the development of drugs to treat a human disease starts with laboratory experiments to identify what are the effects of a discovered compound in living cells, a tissue, or an organ relevant to the disease. If the concept works in the laboratory, the research moves to the preclinical testing phase, usually in animals that have a condition that resembles the human disease, which the drug is aimed to treat. If successful in these animal models, then the research moves further to human testing in clinical trials. Along the entire development process, the benefit from the tested drug is assessed against the risk, and only the drugs that maintain a favorable benefit-to-risk relationship eventually reach the market.

While applying a measured dose of a drug to cells or a tissue in the controlled environment of a laboratory may produce the same result again and again, the studies in humans can produce an astonishing array of expected and unexpected findings. It is because of this variability among humans that clinical studies with a large number of participants are required to test drugs for their clinical benefit (effectiveness) and safety. The drug approval process by regulatory agencies such as the US Food and Drug Administration (FDA) includes detailed review of clinical trial information on drug safety and effectiveness from hundreds, and often thousands, of patients. In the vast majority of cases, even after the drug has been approved, the research continues to gain more details on its safe and beneficial use.

But why am I focusing on the drug development process? A drug's **effectiveness**, which is how well the drug achieves its desired treatment goal, and **its safety**, which is how much damage the drug may cause when it is used to achieve these treatment goals, are the factors that your doctor is going to consider when choosing the appropriate treatment for your condition. I will provide a brief overview on how safety and effectiveness are determined in clinical studies before or after drug approval as well as on the relevance of these concepts to making individual drug-related choices.

Despite the wealth of data on how drugs work and what side effects they cause, in the majority of cases the information we have is on a **group** level. It is virtually impossible to predict fully the desired, and the undesired, effects of a drug in an individual in a manner we might be able to do in a laboratory environment. Giving the same dose of ibuprofen to five people with a headache will not result in the same extent of pain relief in all five; nor will the same dose of insulin to reduce blood sugar (glucose) levels work equally in five diabetic patients. We all belong to the same *Homo sapiens* species—the group level—yet there is an enormous number of factors, or variables, the combination of which will ultimately decide how safe and how effective a given drug is for each one of us.

EFFECTIVENESS: DISEASES, DRUGS, AND INDIVIDUAL RESPONSES

Two patients may share the same diagnosis, but no disease or illness has an identical course in any two individuals. As Sir William Osler (one of the founding professors of Johns Hopkins Hospital) described in 1903, "The problems of disease are much more complicated and difficult than any others with which the trained mind has to grapple; the conditions in any given case may be unlike those in any other; each case, indeed, may have its own problem."

Let's start with a simple example of two members in the same household suffering from a respiratory virus: the common cold. Even if they are siblings, they are probably not going to have exactly the same set of symptoms, same grade of fever, and exact duration of cold. As individuals, we have a different set of genes (unless we are identical twins); the immune system has developed somewhat differently in each one of us based on previous illnesses and environmental exposures; and differences in age and current medical conditions play an important role as well. With the common cold, for example, it may not really matter if your symptoms lasted 3 or 4 days, and the differences among individuals may be of minor importance. But when we are talking about more complex diseases, which involve several systems of the body, the difference between two patients sharing the same diagnosis may be enormous. For example, it is known that long-term diabetes causes impairment in nerve function because of the damage that high blood sugar (glucose) levels can cause to the nervous tissue. However, if you investigate 20 people who have been suffering from diabetes for 15 years each, you may not find even two with the same set of symptoms or the same complaints related to their nerve function impairment. One individual may report symptoms mainly related to damage to nerves that innervate the bowel (resulting in bloating or constipation), another may report symptoms related to reproductive and urinary nervous systems (e.g., erectile dysfunction or urinary incontinence), two others may have mainly different painful symptoms related to damage of the sensory nerves in the skin, and so on. As you can see, various pathological processes of the same disease are likely to take a somewhat different route in different individuals, which will of course be a factor in variability in response to medications. Therefore, a drug that worked for your sister/neighbor/friend may or may not work to the same extent for you.

It is also important to understand how the information (or data) on drug effectiveness is obtained from clinical trials. There exist all sorts of clinical trials; they may differ by design, size, quality, and other parameters—however, the current basis for approving a drug lies in presenting scientific evidence that in a group of patients, on average, the drug was more effective than no treatment (or *placebo* treatment), or it was equally effective to another established treatment.

From that step on, each prescriber uses her or his clinical experience and judgment to "translate" the research findings as they apply to the individual patient. Let's look at an example to illustrate how that happens. Assume that a pharmaceutical company has developed a new drug, NO-TENSION, for treating high blood pressure (hypertension). The company carries out a clinical trial in which 200 patients with hypertension receive the study drug and 200 patients with hypertension receive an inactive pill (placebo) once a day for 6 months. The results of the trial state that in the group of patients that received NO-TENSION, the systolic (upper) blood pressure was reduced by average 22 mm Hg (millimeters of mercury, the unit for measuring blood pressure) after 6 months. In the placebo group, the average reduction in blood pressure over the same time period was 9 mm Hg. The statistical analysis finds that this difference is significant and determines that NO-TENSION reduces blood pressure better than the placebo treatment. Moreover, the researchers find that in the group receiving NO-TENSION, there have been fewer cases of heart attacks than in the control group. The conclusion is that NO-TENSION is an effective drug for treating hypertension.

Does that mean that any person who starts taking NO-TENSION will have his or her blood pressure reduced by 22 mm Hg after 6 months? **Absolutely not!** In fact, maybe none of the patients in the research study had exactly 22 mm Hg reduction in their blood pressure. What the study tells us precisely is that if the drug is prescribed to a group of patients who are similar to those enrolled in the study, there will likely be an average reduction of 22 mm Hg in blood pressure over 6 months. Figure 2.1 shows hypothetical systolic blood pressure measurements of all patients before the study (circles) on the left side, and the measurement of NO-TENSION group (squares) and placebo group (triangles) on the right side. Despite the **average** difference of 13 mm Hg between NO-TENSION and placebo at the end of treatment, it is obvious that some patients in the NO-TENSION group did worse with that those with placebo, and a few even had their blood pressure increased over the course of treatment.

At this point, the individual's response to the prescribed drug becomes important. Some people will respond well to a drug, while

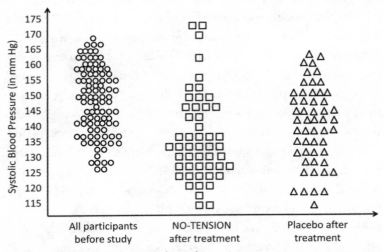

Figure 2.1. Hypothetical systolic (upper) blood pressure measurements in a research study before treatment (*circles*) and after 6 months of treatment with experimental drug (NO-TENSION, *squares*) and inactive placebo (*triangles*). The presumed difference between average values in NO-TENSION and placebo groups is 13 mm Hg.

others will not, for a variety of reasons that I will discuss in detail in Chapters 3 and 4. Unfortunately, many clinical trials cannot provide information detailed enough to predict effectiveness on an individual level. And this is where the clinicians use their judgment and experience to prescribe the best possible treatment for you. But as a patient, it is critical that you understand this variability. You may be the one to get the full benefit of the drug, but you also might eventually be the outlier in the group and not benefit from the drug despite the fact that the drug was approved for treating your condition. This is also one of the reasons your physician may try prescribing several medications (one after another, or in parallel) to find the treatment that is most appropriate for you. The better you understand how each of your drugs work, what the possible range of desirable and undesirable effects is, and how exactly to determine treatment success, the better you can communicate your treatment experience with your physician so that the treatment can be adjusted to maximize its benefit and your safety.

In the book *De Morbis Popularibus,* Hippocrates wrote: "The art (of medicine) consists in three things—the disease, the patient, and the physician. The physician is the servant of the art, and the patient must combat the disease along with the physician" (Latin translation, London, 1717). The coming chapters will provide you with important principles about drug treatment so that you are best equipped with appropriate tools to "combat the disease" together with your team of care providers.

SAFETY: SIDE EFFECTS AND THEIR PREVENTION

The **effectiveness** component outlined in the first part of this chapter is only half of the story. The other half, arguably no less important, is drug **safety**. In the physicians' oath, *Primum non nocere*—"First, do no harm," is one of the fundamental principles of medical ethics and practice. Beyond the fact that you, as a patient, want the drug to treat your condition, you need it to do so without causing you harm.

Let's discuss the same example of hypertension treatment with NO-TENSION. We only discussed the beneficial effects on high blood pressure. If the drug causes undesired effects that are bad enough so that you need to stop the treatment or need to take a lower (and maybe less effective) dose of the drug, this is a serious limitation. Clinical trials would typically report what kind of side effects the study patients experienced and at what frequency (e.g., 10% reported headaches, 15% reported nausea, and 3% had infections) and whether any of these side effects caused patients to drop out of the study. However, it is important to understand that *causality* (that X was a result of Y) is not always established in these cases. If a patient was nauseated during the study, nausea will appear as one of the reported adverse effects, even if it was caused by a stomach virus and not the study drug. But beyond the problems with establishing causality, clinical trial reports often cannot provide detailed information on which patients are more likely to experience undesired effects.

At this point, again, the healthcare professional's clinical judgment and experience are indispensable in determining which dose of which drug is going to be safe for you, although "safe," as it relates to drugs, is quite an ambiguous term and is dependent on context. If you take a drug for a minor headache once in a while—"safe" would probably mean close to zero side effects. For a mild headache, you wouldn't consider a painkiller that may cause hair loss. So, hair loss would be an unacceptable adverse effect in that context. On the other hand, for a drug that has a good chance to treat cancer or a life-threatening infection, hair loss might be a relatively moderate, or acceptable, price to pay, and the drug may be considered "safe" in that context.

I will be discussing the individual variability in response to drugs at many occasions throughout the book, but there is another major safety issue that we need to consider seriously: the chance of human error. In today's fast, ever-growing era of new drugs, data, and technologies, it is practically impossible for one person to keep abreast of all the information required for safe and effective use of medications. Add to it a clinician's long working days, tiredness, and momentary lack of concentration—and the scenario of a medication error is not that unlikely.

When I was in graduate school, I used to do evening and weekend shifts in a community pharmacy. One winter evening, a young couple came in with a prescription for their child. It was a prescription for *ranitidine*—an oral liquid medication to treat reflux (increased acidity in the stomach). The prescribed dose was 8 mL twice a day, and the prescription was from a pediatrician whom I knew and highly respected. I noticed that the baby was 4 weeks old, and as with all pediatric prescriptions, as a pharmacist you routinely double-check the dose to make sure it was correctly adjusted to weight and age.

The baby was born prematurely, and at the age of 4 weeks she still weighed 6.5 pounds (3 kilograms). The usual dose of ranitidine is around 2 milligrams per kilogram body weight every 8 to 12 hours, which for that baby meant 6 mg per dose. The prescribed syrup contains 15 mg of *ranitidine* in each 1 mL, which means that 8 mL (in the prescription) would result in 120 mg (and not 6 mg) of the drug per dose. I called the physician's office—it was 7:30 p.m., and I could tell by the secretary's voice that it has been a hell of a day in the clinic. She politely asked me to wait a bit because the doctor was seeing the last child of that day, 1.5 hours after his clinic was supposed to be closed. During our conversation, the pediatrician realized that he meant to prescribe 8 drops per dose, but wrote 8 mL. Usually, 1 mL contains about 20 drops, so 8 drops would indeed be an appropriate dose. But if the baby received 8 mL, she would get a dose 20 times higher than intended.

Imagine that as an adult you are prescribed an antibiotic and instead of two pills twice a day you are instructed to take 40 pills twice a day. Forty pills would be of course an unreasonable amount of medicine for an adult, but the parents among you would agree that a dose of 8 mL (less than 2 teaspoons) does not sound like an alarming amount for a 4-week old baby and could have easily gone unnoticed, with potentially serious consequences. This time, we all got lucky, and the baby received her intended dose of 8 drops. But my point is that errors may be made, even by the best and most thorough professionals. You might think that what I described previously was a once-in-a-lifetime slip, but the statistics suggest otherwise. The "To Err Is Human" report of the Institute of Medicine concluded that 48,000 to 96,000 people die every year in US hospitals because of medical errors, with adverse drug effects being among the most common causes of death. And these errors occur at all levels, from patient identification to prescribing, dispensing, administering, and monitoring. The full picture might be even more disturbing because the previous numbers do not include cases occurring outside of hospitals and cases in which people have been injured but survived. It is true that some of these patients died because of unexpected side effects; nevertheless, the report concludes that a substantial number of in-hospital deaths could have been **prevented**.

Without blaming a specific factor or system, we should first face the facts that medication errors happen, that they happen much more frequently that we think or would like them to happen, and that they can result in serious consequences to our health. And there is no reason to believe that outside the hospital setting, the picture is any different. Patients at home may be less sick and less fragile, but on the other hand, many aspects of their therapy are not under direct supervision of trained health professionals.

Many hospitals and clinics make an enormous effort to improve the safety of their operation, but the system is still far from being error-proof. Always assume that an error is possible; it might not be very likely, but it is possible. Your healthcare providers will do their best to give you the appropriate drug, at the appropriate dose, for the appropriate duration. They will stay late at work to double-check your medical record and write an accurate visit summary and plan, they will stay awake late reading to learn more about your condition, and they will do additional fellowships and take continuing education courses to improve their knowledge on treating your diseases. But we are talking about **your** health—and the stakes are the highest for **you**. **You** are an essential part of the team that treats you—throw in your best effort to make sure that your treatment is appropriate and to avoid being on the receiving end of a medication error.

THE FIVE ESSENTIAL ELEMENTS OF DRUG SAFETY

Taking into account the patient variability and the risk for errors presented in this chapter, the **general approach** for safe drug prescribing should include at least the following five elements, which I consider essential:

1. Healthcare professionals should prescribe drugs within the limits of their competence. Although any doctor can lawfully prescribe virtually any drug, research shows that competence and experience within the practice scope matters. *Make your treatment safer by having the medications for your disease prescribed by a relevant specialist, rather than a physician whose scope of practice only marginally deals with your conditions.*

2. The prescribed drug should not be known to worsen any of your conditions or organ functions and should not be administered if you have allergies to the drug. For example, if the prescribed drug may cause kidney damage, and your kidney function is already impaired, the drug may be particularly dangerous for you. *Let your doctor know about all your medical conditions and allergies. Study your new drugs to understand their potential risks.*

3. The prescribed drug should not negatively affect or be affected by (in other words, interact with) other drugs, vitamins, or supplements you take. *Always consult your doctor or pharmacist regarding the compatibility of any new prescription or over-the-counter drug with the list of your other medications.*

4. The dosage and the duration of treatment should be appropriate for your condition and age. *Verify with your prescriber or the pharmacist the strength and the amount of daily doses you should take as well as the recommended duration of treatment and any special considerations concerning your age.*

5. Patients should be aware of serious adverse effects of each of their drugs, understand how to identify these, and have practical recommendations on "what to do if." This is a major safety issue. *Ask your physician to outline clearly the dangerous side effects of each of your drugs and make sure you know how to recognize these effects. Have a clear plan for taking the appropriate action if you suspect you are experiencing a dangerous side effect.*

Providing your physician with accurate information about your allergies, previous experiences with drugs, information about your kidney and liver function, any diseases you may have, and drugs (prescription, over the counter, or illicit) that you have been taking will reduce the chance of missing one of these criteria and will increase the likelihood of safe prescribing. The same goes for reporting any undesired effect you may be experiencing since taking a new drug. It is ultimately your responsibility as a patient to be a partner in your medication management, to be attentive to your own body, and to provide relevant feedback to the provider.

Take-Home Message

Your doctors, nurses, and other healthcare professionals are all trained to prevent and treat your diseases. But you are different from someone else with the same diagnosis, and your feedback and proper communication with your doctor can prevent undesired consequences and improve the desired results of your treatment. However, for this useful communication to occur, it is important that you understand the general principles of safe and effective drug therapy and the specific details about the medications you take. Your response to a drug may be somewhat different compared with another person's, and being mindful of these differences can help reduce the potential for medication errors.

[3]

WHAT DOES OUR BODY DO
TO DRUGS?

The Amazing Journey of a Molecule

Any drug you take will follow a certain path in your body to reach the organ(s) where it is active. It will also undergo a series of steps that ensure the drug eventually leaves your body. Becoming familiar with these processes will help you understand how your body handles drug molecules; how they reach, for example, your brain or your heart; and how changes in your health, or starting a new medication, can affect the safety and the effectiveness of drugs you take.

You (and your prescriber) are only interested in very specific effects of each of your drugs in treating your medical condition. If you need a treatment for rapid heartbeat, you are only interested in the drug's action on slowing down the contractions of your heart muscle. If the drug also slowed down your intestine and caused constipation, most of us would consider this an undesired or adverse effect. But it's important to realize that this is a conscious expectation for good and bad effects of a drug. Unlike our mind, though, our body does not have a preference for desired or undesired effects of drugs, nor can it differentiate between them. Actually, the human body does not recognize most drugs as useful molecules at all. With the exception of a few hormones such as insulin or testosterone, there is not much our body can do with drugs for its own utility purposes. Most drugs are not useful for producing energy or building DNA and therefore are treated by our body as alien, foreign compounds. Hundreds of thousands of years of evolution have taught the human organism to get rid of foreign nonessential molecules to avoid poisoning, and to do so as quickly as possible.

From the moment a drug enters the body, whether as a pill, an injection, a rectal suppository, or by any other route, it will undergo a series of processes such that it can eventually be eliminated from the body. The scientific discipline that studies this movement of drugs in the body is called **pharmacokinetics** (from Greek: *pharmakon*—drug, substance; and *kinetikos*—movement).

Pharmacokinetics can be described by four processes that each drug undergoes within a body: *absorption, distribution, metabolism,* and *excretion* (abbreviated as ADME), and this chapter will describe these four processes step by step. The familiarity with ADME principles is instrumental for understanding many of the individual differences in drug response, many of the reasons drug therapies fail, and many of the incompatibilities or interactions among drugs. This chapter is somewhat more "technical" than others but will focus mainly on terms that are important for understanding the subsequent chapters. I encourage you to do your best to read it because it covers key principles that will increase your overall understanding of how drugs work.

ABSORPTION

Absorption is the process by which the drug reaches the bloodstream after you take it. The absorption process occurs regardless if you took the drug orally, inhaled to the airway, or injected under the skin, although it would be somewhat different in each of these cases. Sometimes we desire a local effect from a drug (e.g., using an antibiotic ointment for a skin infection, or injecting a steroid medication into an inflamed joint), and in these cases we are interested in minimal absorption of the drug to the bloodstream. But more often, like with drugs taken as pills or injected under the skin, we want the drug to reach the bloodstream (also called the *systemic circulation*) because it is through blood that the drug can be further carried to the organ we want it to reach, such as the brain, the kidneys, or the heart. Unless I specifically refer to a local treatment, most of this book will describe the more common, *systemic* treatments that require that the drug enters the bloodstream to reach its target organ(s).

The absorption process is irrelevant when the drug is injected intravenously (IV) directly into the blood because all 100% of the drug reaches the bloodstream, with no variability between individuals. But when the drug is administered by mouth (*orally*), the fraction, or proportion, of the dose that eventually reaches the bloodstream can vary. This fraction can be as high as nearly 100% for some drugs, when the entire drug dose eventually reaches the bloodstream, or as low as zero for other drugs, when none of the drug reaches the bloodstream. It can also be anything in-between.

First, let me describe the normal absorption process, which will later allow me to focus on individual differences in drug absorption and possible treatment challenges associated with it. I will focus on oral absorption (when the drug is taken by mouth) because this is the most common way of taking medications.

Gastrointestinal Sites of Absorption

When you swallow a pill, it goes down the *esophagus* (Figure 3.1) and reaches the stomach, which has an acidic environment. In that

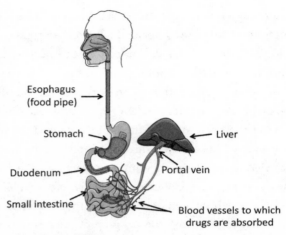

Esophagus
(food pipe)

Stomach

Liver

Duodenum

Portal vein

Small intestine

Blood vessels to which
drugs are absorbed

Figure 3.1. Key sections of the gastrointestinal (GI) tract relevant for drug absorption after oral intake. Absorption occurs when drugs cross the lining of the GI tract (from inside to outside) and enter the blood vessels, which carry the drug with the bloodstream to the liver. Credit: Elements for this image obtained from Servier image bank: http://www.servier.com/Powerpoint-image-bank.

environment, the pill (whether a capsule or a tablet) breaks down and dissolves in the stomach fluid so that single molecules of the drug now "float" in this fluid. Unless the drug is broken down to the level of single molecules, it won't get absorbed in to the bloodstream. For most medications, this breakdown process may take 20 to 40 minutes, depending on the type of pill and the stomach contents. If you take the medication in a liquid form (e.g., syrup), it will dissolve faster because the breakdown process of a tablet is skipped. Some drug products are designed not to release their content immediately but instead to do so in a modified or controlled fashion. These drugs may undergo a somewhat different absorption process, as I will discuss in Chapter 5.

When the drug is dissolved, it needs to either pass through the stomach wall or go down further to the small intestine and pass through the intestine wall in order to get to the blood vessels located on the outer side of the *gastrointestinal* (GI) tract. The intestine wall serves as a sort of a filter to prevent some unnecessary or toxic compounds from reaching the bloodstream.

The blood from these GI blood vessels is drained to a single vein called the *portal vein*, which enters the liver. The liver is capable of breaking down and neutralizing many chemical substances, especially those foreign to our body. This absorption pathway, which "routes" the drugs to the liver first, ensures that everything we eat or drink also gets filtered by the liver before reaching the rest of the organs (heart, lungs, brain). This process of "double filtration" is common to all mammals and is in place from the evolutionary standpoint to decrease the harm from poisons or toxins that were unintentionally digested. It is only after the drug molecules leave the liver that they reach the general bloodstream for the first time.

Very few drugs are substantially absorbed directly through the stomach, and those that do typically result in a quick effect. Alcohol, for example, gets absorbed through the stomach, and may reach high blood levels within 10 to 15 minutes in some individuals. The majority of orally taken drugs, on the contrary, will not have full effects in the 10- to 15-minute time frame. Most drugs need to pass further down to the *small intestine* to be absorbed to the bloodstream. From the stomach, drugs pass down first to the upper part of the small intestine, called the *duodenum,* and then further down the rest of the small intestine.

Knowing which part of the intestine your drug absorbs from can help you understand the timing of the drug's effect. Drugs remain in the stomach for about 30 minutes, then they take about 3 hours to pass through the small intestine and approximately 24 hours to pass through the large intestine. These times can be affected by food intake and by different conditions such as diarrhea (that would shorten them) or diabetes (that would prolong them).

Mechanisms that Can Affect Drug Absorption

The human body has two absorption barriers, or filters: the *intestine wall barrier* and the *liver barrier*. The intestine wall is built from cells that are tightly bound to each other along the whole intestine. The drug needs to navigate across these cells (or between the cells in some cases) to reach the other side of the intestine wall and enter the vessels that carry blood from the intestine to the liver. A number of processes that take place in this little encounter between drug molecules and intestine wall cells (called *enterocytes*) may either reduce the amount of drug that is eventually absorbed to the bloodstream or block the absorption process altogether. The two key barriers here are *enzymes* and *efflux pumps*. There are certain proteins (called *enzymes*) inside these enterocytes whose role is to identify molecules foreign to the body and to break them down. Most drugs will be broken down to some extent by these enzymes. In addition to this enzyme barrier, there are *efflux pumps*—proteins located on the surface of the enterocyte that simply take the "intruder" molecule and pump it out of the intestine wall back to the hollow part of the intestine. These *efflux pumps* are another mechanism of defense against poisons and foreign substances.

The proportion of the drug that passed the intestine wall barrier will reach the *portal vein*, where the blood will carry the drug into the liver—which is the second absorption barrier. The liver contains similar enzymes, which can further break down the drug. Eventually, the *percentage* of drug that reaches the *bloodstream* after passing through the intestine wall absorption barriers and the liver barrier is referred to as *drug bioavailability*.

The reason I am mentioning the term *bioavailability* is that it is important in determining the extent to which the effectiveness of your medication can be affected in different circumstances. Let's say you took a pill that contains 100 mg of a drug, 75% of which was broken down in the intestine and the liver by the previously mentioned enzymes, so that eventually 25 mg reached your bloodstream. In this case the drug had 25% bioavailability (because only 25 mg of the 100 mg that you took is going to affect you and result in any desired or undesired effects). Now imagine a situation in which these "defensive barriers" in the intestine and the liver are affected by a disease or another drug and fail to work. In this scenario, all 100 mg of the drug may be absorbed to the bloodstream—which is likely to result in 4 times the amount of its effects. It would be like taking a quadruple dose of the drug under normal conditions. While for some drugs it may not make a huge difference, for other drugs this can be fatal. In subsequent chapters, I will discuss what specific conditions and drugs might lead to the failure of these defensive barriers, and thus result in enhanced effect or toxicity of some drugs.

To summarize this section: drugs that are administered in ways other than directly into the vein undergo an absorption process, which will eventually determine what proportion of the drug is available to exert its action. This proportion is called a drug's bioavailability. The transfer processes through intestine wall and the liver are the major determinants of oral drug bioavailability and can substantially influence the desired and undesired effects of your medications.

DISTRIBUTION

After your drug has overcome the absorption hurdle and reached the bloodstream, it undergoes a *distribution* process via the bloodstream throughout body organs and tissues. As I mentioned previously, we may want the drug to go only to a specific organ, for example, to the heart. However, in most cases this is beyond our control, and the drug will be carried by the bloodstream to reach each organ based on the drug's physical and chemical properties.

It would have been simple if "adding" a drug to the body was like adding a drug to a glass of water. If you add 100 units of a drug to a glass with 100 mL water and stir until it dissolves, you will get an even distribution of the drug in the water, with *concentration* of 1 unit in each 1 mL of the liquid (solution) anywhere in the glass—whether you sample at the top or at the bottom. The picture is different with the whole body, though, because the blood flow rate to various organs is different, and organs differ in their composition, size, and structure. After the drug has reached the bloodstream, it is the **distribution** process that will determine how much of the drug each organ gets, which is critical for determining the extent of desired and undesired effects of the drug. Higher distribution = more effect; lower distribution = less effect.

General Considerations in Drug Distribution

There are, in fact, enormous differences in distribution properties among the various drugs because they do not reach all organs in the same amount. For example, if your heart weighs ¾ pound (320 grams) and your brain weighs 4 times more—it does not mean that your brain will receive 4 times more drug than your heart. Some drugs, such as *digoxin* for the treatment of heart failure, will reach 5 to 10 times **lower** concentration in the brain than in blood but 50 times **higher** concentration in the heart; other drugs, such as *diphenhydramine* (Benadryl, others) for the treatment of allergy, will reach a 10 times **higher** concentration in the brain than in the blood. Because of these different distribution properties, we may commonly experience side effects unrelated to the drug's main desired activity. For example, we may take *diphenhydramine* (Benadryl) to treat an allergy or nasal congestion, but because of its enhanced brain distribution properties, the drug reaches the brain and acts on certain nerve cells to cause sleepiness and drowsiness—which have nothing to do with the antiallergic effect of the drug.

There are a variety of factors that determine the distribution properties of each drug, but two of the most important properties in this regard are (1) whether the drug molecule prefers to be in an aqueous environment (a compound like *table salt* that can be dissolved in water) or in a fatty environment (a compound like *vitamin D* that will not dissolve in water but can be dissolved in oil), and (2) whether the drug is caught by *efflux pumps* (which I mentioned with regard to absorption in the gut, but these pumps exist in other organs as well).

Water-soluble, or *hydrophilic*, drugs (from *hydro*—water, and *philos*—attracted; i.e., attracted to water) will typically prefer staying in the bloodstream and urine rather than traveling to organs with high lipid (fat) content like brain, skin, or fat tissue. These kinds of water-soluble drugs, for example, can be very useful in treating blood diseases and urinary tract disorders, where we need to achieve high blood or urine concentration without affecting other organs much. On the other hand, *lipophilic* drugs (*lipos*—fat, i.e., attracted to fat) will typically readily concentrate in fatty tissues and also in the brain. The reason that lipophilic drugs are attracted to the brain is that most nerves are covered by a myelin sheath, which increases the speed by which impulses are conducted. Myelin is a fatty substance and is a major contributor to the fact that about 60% of human brain consists of fat (or lipids, to be more accurate).

The brain, however, is the most protected organ in the sense of drug distribution because it has some effective mechanisms for preventing the penetration of foreign molecules. The main defense mechanism is called the *blood-brain barrier*, which all molecules must overcome in order to reach the brain from the bloodstream. The *blood-brain barrier* works similarly to the intestinal absorption barrier but is less "penetrable." It consists of cells that have different kinds of *efflux pumps* that identify foreign molecules and throw these back into the bloodstream, preventing their entry to the brain. As you will see in future chapters, some drugs may affect the *blood-brain barrier* and thus decrease or increase the brain distribution of certain medications.

Factors Affecting Drug Distribution

Certain conditions can greatly affect drug distribution, such as pregnancy or significant changes in weight or muscle mass. We need to be aware of these because a change in drug concentration in one organ or tissue may significantly change its concentration elsewhere in the body and affect its desired or undesired effects. I will give you a few examples to provide a better understanding how changes in your body can affect drug distribution and therefore drug effectiveness and safety.

Let us imagine that Angela, a 132-pound (60-kg) woman, is taking *hormonosterol* (fake name) for a long period of time, a drug for which the proportion of its *fat-to-blood distribution* is **9 to 1**. Let's for a second disregard the other body parts and assume that *hormonosterol* is a female hormone that requires a certain blood concentration in order to exert its action. In this scenario, if Angela takes a 100-mg pill, 90 mg of *hormonosterol* will go to fat tissue and 10 mg will go to blood. Now let's imagine that Angela gained 26 lb (12 kg) over the recent year. It is a 20% gain in total weight, but if the gained weight all comes from fat and not muscles, her fat mass may have increased by 50%. With this change, the new distribution ratio of *hormonosterol* will be roughly **14 to 1 (because the amount of fat increased by additional 50%)**. What this change means is that of the 100-mg drug Angela takes, 93.3 mg will now go to fat and 6.7 mg will remain in blood. The consequence is that Angela will lose about one third of the effective drug concentration in the blood (from 10 mg to 6.7 mg), which could result in a loss of the drug's effectiveness.

This situation of drug distribution will differ a lot from a drug to drug, based on some of the lipophilic and hydrophilic properties we discussed previously. If Angela were to take a more *hydrophilic* drug, for which the fat-to-blood ratio is **1 to 9** (and not **9 to 1** as for *hormonosterol*), it would not be affected much by her weight gain. Therefore, the doses of certain drugs may be based on the patient's weight (e.g., in milligrams of drug per kilogram of body weight), rather than as a fixed adult dose. This weight-based dose adjustment can allow more accurate "tailoring" of drug effects.

In reality, drugs are distributed to all different body compartments. From the bloodstream, the drug reaches many tissues: the brain, muscles, bones, liver, kidney, nerves, blood cells, and others. The road to safe and effective drug treatment passes through understanding the conditions that can change the distribution of a drug to certain compartments. With that knowledge we would be able to better predict the desired and undesired drug effects. My goal is not to make you experts in drug distribution but to provide some background so that examples given later in the book make sense.

To summarize this section: when the drug reaches the bloodstream, there are a variety of factors that will determine the amount of drug that each of the organs will get. Since the concentration of the drug at each site is going to determine its desired and undesired effects, you should be aware of the fact that various conditions can change the distribution ratios of the drugs, which can result in increased or decreased effects. The examples that were provided are aimed to illustrate that the same change, such as weight gain, may change the effect of one drug but not necessarily another.

METABOLISM

Metabolism is the main process by which most drugs lose their effect over time. Metabolism is synonymous to *breakdown*, and for the majority of drugs it occurs in the **liver**—within cells called *hepatocytes* (from Greek: *hepat*—liver; and *kytos*—cell). Imagine that every time a drug is carried with the bloodstream through the liver, a certain proportion of it undergoes *breakdown*; this process occurs again and again until no drug is left in the bloodstream. While the liver is the main metabolizing organ, it is worth noting that drugs can be broken down (metabolized) at other sites as well, including the intestine, the lungs, the bloodstream, and even in the placenta of a pregnant woman.

But let's get back to the liver. The main breakdown of drugs is performed by a group of enzymes called **cytochrome P-450** (or **CYP**) enzymes. CYP enzymes make permanent changes in the drug structure to make it inactive and help our body get rid of it, although in some cases the products of breakdown may have certain activity.

To reiterate, the liver is one of the most important organs responsible for drug breakdown. It is important to remember that diseases that affect the liver can have a substantial effect on drug pharmacokinetics. Let's take an example to illustrate how that may be occurring. Cecilia is healthy, and her liver breaks down 50% of drug M in 12 hours. Now Cecilia has contracted hepatitis, which affects her liver, and her sick liver "works" only at half of the previous capacity. In this situation, Cecilia's liver will break down only 25% of the drug in 12 hours. This means that when she takes her next dose of drug M, it will have a larger effect because it will build up on top of a higher amount of drug M remaining unmetabolized in her body. If this repetitive dosing continues, the amount of the drug in Cecilia's body is likely to keep increasing over the following few days and lead to undesired or toxic effects. A similar process may occur if Cecilia's liver is healthy, but she has now started taking another drug X that affects the liver's ability to break down drug M. This may happen, for example, if drug X interferes with the activity of CYP enzymes. Taking both drugs M and X will cause a "drug-drug interaction"—meaning that one drug (X) will influence the other drug's (M) action. Drug-drug interactions are a separate area of interest, which I will discuss in more detail in Chapter 8.

Genetic Differences in Drug Metabolism

One level of complexity causing different individuals to respond differently to the same drug is the fact that not all CYP enzymes work at the same rate in all people. Our genetic makeup will determine how the various CYPs work. For example, one of the CYP enzymes, called CYP 2D6, which is responsible for breaking down many painkillers, psychiatric drugs, and heart medications, does not function properly in some people. These people would be called "poor metabolizers" of that particular CYP enzyme. If you are a *poor metabolizer* and take a drug that is metabolized by that CYP enzyme, the drug will be broken down less effectively and thus can accumulate within your body (an outcome similar to the previous scenario of Cecilia and hepatitis).

There are also substantial ethnic differences in the activity of CYP enzymes. For example, in the Caucasian population, one of every 15 people is a *poor metabolizer* of CYP 2D6, while in Asian (Thai, Chinese, Japanese) populations, only one of 100 people is a poor metabolizer of 2D6. For another major enzyme involved in drug metabolism, called CYP 2C19, the ethnic picture is quite the opposite—one of every five Asian individuals is a *poor metabolizer* of CYP 2C19, while only one of every 50 Caucasians is a *poor metabolizer*. There are tests available to determine some of these genetic differences. While these tests are not used routinely, they are sometimes performed for safer prescribing of certain drugs such as warfarin or clopidogrel for blood thinning (see Chapter 13). These genetic tests can be also ordered for individuals who display unexpected responses to drugs or are at high risk for developing serious side effects.

Some healthcare professionals among pharmacists, doctors, and nurses are well trained in analyzing these complex issues of drug metabolism. In addition, there are books, software, and online resources available to assist in the process. The main challenge is that many patients with complex drug regimens do not have their medication therapy assessed thoroughly and reassessed when a change occurs in their treatment or in the function of their various organs. This kind of a comprehensive drug review is something that I would highly recommend to any person taking more than a few chronic medications.

To summarize this section: drugs undergo various breakdown (metabolism) processes, which mainly occur in the liver by enzymes that belong to the cytochrome P-450 (CYP) family. These metabolic processes usually inactivate drugs (although more rarely can turn an inactive drug to an active one). Some drugs, diseases, and our genetic makeup may affect the rate of drug breakdown. It is important to have a formal assessment of medication therapy on a regular basis to avoid problems and underdosing or overdosing due to changes in liver function or significant drug-drug interactions.

EXCRETION

Excretion is a combination of processes by which the drugs are eliminated (cleared) from the body. Some drugs are excreted unchanged, "as is," and some are broken down to fragments following metabolism, and these fragments are excreted later. Our body gets rid of most drugs through feces or urine, although some drugs undergo unique processes and leave the body in another manner, for example, through the lungs.

A drug may have several routes of excretion. For example, 40% of the dose may be excreted into the urine through the kidneys, and 60% may undergo metabolism by the liver. In most *healthy* people, the overall time it takes to get rid of a particular drug is quite similar. Each drug has a characteristic *half-life*—which is a measure of how fast the drug is going to disappear from the body. The longer the half-life, the slower the excretion (disappearing) process. After about five half-lives, more than 95% of the drug has disappeared from your bloodstream. For example, if you read that a drug you take has a half-life of 4 hours, it means that 24 hours after you took a single dose, there will very little drug left in your body.

There are several parameters responsible for differences in drug excretion among individuals—factors such as kidney function and liver function, certain medical conditions, age, and the use of other medications. Excretion through *urine* is indeed the more common route of drug excretion, and kidney function plays an important role in a person's ability to get rid of the drugs and their metabolites. For example, if you take a drug that is excreted only by kidneys and now your kidneys work at 50% capacity because of a disease, it may take twice as long to get rid of the drug, and in this situation the drug dose needs to be reduced so that it does not cause undesired effects.

To summarize this section: excretion is the process (or combination of processes) by which the drug leaves the body. In healthy individuals it is somewhat predictable because the information on metabolism, elimination, and other pharmacokinetic parameters is available at the time of drug approval. But as I mentioned, based on the function of various organs and the intake of certain drugs, the excretion of a drug may change, which will affect its concentration in the blood and therefore its effectiveness and side effects.

Take-Home Message

Absorption, distribution, metabolism, and excretion (ADME) processes are complex, but this is invariably what happens to each drug
we take. Having a reasonable grasp on the four ADME principles of
drug pharmacokinetics will allow having a clear picture of what your
body does with drugs when you take them. Understanding these
concepts is helpful in asking relevant questions about how certain
foods, diseases, or drugs are going to affect the desired and undesired
effects of your medications.

[4]

WHAT DO THE DRUGS DO
TO OUR BODY?

In contrast to pharmacokinetics, which explains what the body does to the drug, I will now explore what the drug does to the body, or how drugs actually work. The discipline that covers this topic is called pharmacodynamics (from Greek φάρμακον *(phármakon)*— drug, substance; and δύναμις *(dynamis)*—force, power) and explains the effect of drugs on the body. Understanding how your drugs engage with their targets (receptors) and what systems they activate or block will help you understand and appropriately address the desired and undesired effects of your drugs.

DRUG TARGETS

As I mentioned in Chapter 1 when referring to *drug receptor theory*: drugs typically bind to certain receptors to exert their activity. Only a handful of drugs act in a way that is not mediated by receptors, like, for example, antacids that neutralize the acidity in the stomach and certain laxatives that retain water in the intestine to help treat constipation.

Most drugs simply mimic, enhance, or block the physiological activity of *endogenous* molecules, which are molecules that are produced by (and are present in) our body. There are several types of such *endogenous* molecules, the receptors for which modern drugs target. Let's look at some of the main examples:

1. **Hormones.** Hormones are signaling chemical substances (molecules) produced by various glands in our body and excreted to the bloodstream. For example, *insulin* (discussed in detail in Chapter 14) is a hormone produced by the pancreas gland. After we eat and our blood glucose (sugar) increases, the pancreas releases insulin, which will bind to the *insulin receptor* in various tissues, to move glucose from the blood to organs that need glucose as an energy source. Other examples of hormones include *thyroid hormones* produced by the thyroid gland (see Chapter 19), *testosterone* produced by the testes, and *estrogen* produced by the ovaries.

2. **Neurotransmitters.** Neurotransmitters are also signaling molecules, but they are not released to the bloodstream. Instead, neurotransmitters are released from a nerve and mediate (facilitate) a signal from that nerve to a closely located tissue such as a muscle or another nerve. For example, if you want to close your fingers in a fist, your brain gives a signal to certain nerve cells to release the neurotransmitter *acetylcholine* to the junction between the nerves and the muscles in your hand. By binding to an acetylcholine receptor in the muscles, the neurotransmitter acetylcholine will facilitate muscle flexion to close your fingers. Other examples of neurotransmitters include *serotonin,* which binds to a variety of serotonin receptors and has a critical role in depression (see Chapter 17); *dopamine,* which binds to dopamine receptors and has a critical role in Parkinson's disease and a

variety of mental disorders such as schizophrenia; and *noradrenaline* (synonymous to norepinephrine), which can bind to *adrenergic* receptors and has an important role in asthma (see Chapter 15) and in controlling blood pressure (see Chapter 11). Interestingly, some substances can act as hormones and neurotransmitters, depending on where they are produced. *Noradrenaline* (norepinephrine) acts as a neurotransmitter when it is produced and released by the nerve fibers to act on neighboring nerves, but it acts as a hormone when produced by the adrenal gland (located above the kidneys) and released into the bloodstream.

3. **Growth factors.** Growth factors are usually proteins or steroid hormones that bind to cells (through growth factor receptors) to promote cell growth and maturation. *Nerve growth factor* (NGF) and *erythropoietin* (EPO) are examples of such growth factors. Since anomalies of cell growth and maturation create the basis of many tumors, a variety of cancer treatments target growth factors and their receptors.

4. **Enzymes.** Enzymes are proteins produced by the various cells to assist (catalyze) biochemical processes such as building or breaking down essential molecules like carbohydrates, lipids, neurotransmitters, and proteins (including receptors, hormones, and other enzymes). Since enzymes can affect the activity of many *endogenous* substances, including hormones and neurotransmitters, many drugs target enzymes. Angiotensin-converting enzyme (ACE) inhibitors (see Chapter 11) and monoamine oxidase (MAO) inhibitors (see Chapter 17) are two of the many examples of drug classes targeting enzymes as their receptor target.

5. **DNA and various factors in DNA synthesis.** DNA (deoxyribonucleic acid) carries the genetic information of the human organism and is required for the majority of essential

functions of human cells and for their division and growth. DNA serves as a master template for two main processes: (a) DNA replication, whereby a new copy of the DNA is synthesized for creating every new cell in our body; and (b) protein synthesis, whereby the DNA "master template" is used for creating a molecule called RNA based on which proteins are synthesized. DNA replication and protein synthesis are complex processes controlled in the cell by a variety of transcription factors and other molecules. These transcription factors and components of the DNA itself act as receptors for a variety of endogenous molecules and are also receptors for many drugs that may target DNA replication and processes of protein synthesis.

One thing to keep in mind is that a variety of receptors, hormones, and neurotransmitters can be involved in the pathology of a single disease. Therefore, several treatment possibilities may be available, aiming either to correct the underlying pathology or to treat symptoms associated with the disease. Your physician may have an "arsenal" of potential drugs to prescribe for your condition. Understanding which component of the disease process each of your drugs targets and how each drug works for improving your condition can be instrumental for your safety.

In *Parkinson's disease*, for example, the symptoms are related to a deficit of the neurotransmitter *dopamine* in a certain area of the brain because dopamine-producing nerve cells in that particular region are diseased and eventually die. This pathology results in a variety of symptoms, including tremor (shaky hands) and slow movements. Several treatment options with medications are available; most will be aimed either at increasing the concentration of dopamine in the brain to compensate for lack of sufficient production or at attempting to directly improve the patient's symptoms. You may be prescribed three different drugs: one delivering more dopamine to the brain, as a drug; the second blocking the enzyme that breaks down dopamine in the nervous system to allow longer activity of dopamine that is already produced; and the third treating the tremor without affecting dopamine, by targeting another neurotransmitter. Understanding the role of each of the drugs and the way they work to treat your condition will allow you to better recognize problems with your treatment and better adhere to your physician's instructions and eventually will help you guide your treatment for achieving better outcomes.

AGONISTS AND ANTAGONISTS

Most drugs will bind to one (or more) of the five receptor targets listed previously, and there are two major ways that drug molecules act.

One is by **activating** the receptor, or mimicking what the endogenous substance would do. For example, the placenta of a pregnant woman produces an estrogen-like hormone that binds to receptors in the ovaries to inform the ovary that the woman is now pregnant and does not need the ovary to produce eggs (ovulate). This is the physiological mechanism that prevents menstrual cycles during pregnancy. Oral contraceptive pills are based on hormones that **activate** the same receptors and thus "cheat" the ovary to stop ovulating, despite lack of pregnancy. In this case the drug mimics the *endogenous* substance and is called an **agonist**.

The second major way that drugs interact with receptors is by **blocking** them. In this case, the drug will **prevent** the endogenous substance from binding to the receptor to exert its action. For example, the *endogenous* substances *adrenaline* and *noradrenaline* bind to certain receptors in the heart (called **beta-adrenergic receptors**) and by activating them increase your heart rate and blood pressure. It is through these beta-adrenergic receptors that a release of *adrenaline* causes your heart to beat rapidly when you exercise or are anxious. A group of drugs called **beta-blockers** (or **beta antagonists;** see Chapter 11) act on these beta-adrenergic receptors, but instead of activating as in the case with agonists, they block them, so that when your body releases adrenaline or noradrenaline, it cannot increase your heart rate and blood pressure as much as before because the drug is blocking this effect. These drugs are called **blockers** or **antagonists.**

Pharmacology and pharmacodynamics in particular explore the physiological processes that occur in cells, tissues, and organs after the drug binds to their receptors. This is a huge scientific discipline that covers hundreds of mechanisms involving thousands of biochemical processes. This chapter is not going to touch on the various processes of what is called "signal transduction"—that is, what happens from the moment that a drug binds to its receptor until the final desired effect (e.g., decrease in heart rate) is achieved. Quite honestly, extensive knowledge of physiology and pharmacology is required to process and understand *signal transduction* information in a meaningful manner. In this book, I will try to keep things relatively simple and will refer to the final effect of a drug after binding to the receptor, deliberately skipping the processes that occur "in-between."

DRUG EFFECTS FOLLOWING
THE INTERACTION WITH THE RECEPTORS

The process of the drug's engagement with its appropriate receptor will usually define the drug's "mechanism of action," which is how a drug is known to exert its therapeutic (desired) effect. However, you must also understand that biological systems are rather complex, and it is rare for one drug to bind to only one target and result in only one effect. For example, the *adrenergic* receptors I mentioned earlier are located not only in the heart, and the estrogen receptors are also involved in processes other than ovulation. Often the same types of receptors are located in different tissues or organs. Because of distribution processes described in Chapter 3, we often cannot deliberately guide the drug to reach one tissue while avoiding another tissue, which may result in a drug having several effects. Let's look at how that works: the *adrenergic* receptors (for adrenaline and noradrenaline), in addition to their existence in the heart, are also located on blood vessels where their activation causes narrowing of blood vessels, and in the airway where their activation results in widening of the airway. Consequently, if you are given adrenaline or adrenaline-like drugs, this will result not only in an increase in your heart rate but also in narrowing of blood vessels, which can lead to an increase in blood pressure and to a widening of airway muscles that, for example, can help reduce asthma symptoms.

These additional effects may be desirable or undesirable, depending on the situation. For someone with low blood pressure, this effect on the blood vessels may be beneficial; for another person with high blood pressure, it may be harmful. Accordingly, we may call it either a *therapeutic effect* or an *adverse effect* (a side effect). But the drug does not have sentiments and does not know which effect we are looking for; it simply binds to the receptor it can fit into by the key-and-lock principle and acts either by activating or blocking the receptor. With the knowledge of physiology and information on where each type of receptor is located, clinicians can predict some of these additional desired and undesired effects of drugs before they are prescribed.

Another scenario, typically a less predictable one, is when a drug binds to a receptor it was not designed to bind to. Drugs are molecules, and they typically bind to a receptor by a certain part of the molecule that "fits" the receptor structure (Figure 4.1).

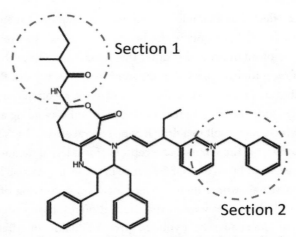

Figure 4.1. Example of a hypothetical drug molecule, which can bind to a certain receptor with one part of its structure (section 1) and to another receptor with a different part of its structure (section 2).

Assume that the molecule in Figure 4.1 was designed to bind to receptor A with its section 1, and does so well. In addition, it was later discovered that it can also bind to a different receptor B with its section 2. This "additional" binding may be completely unanticipated, and then the drug can activate or block an entirely different system and cause **unexpected** side effects. Let's look at an example: a drug that is meant to treat depression by enhancing the activity of the neurotransmitter **serotonin** may cause dry mouth because it "unintentionally" blocks the activity of another neurotransmitter, **acetylcholine,** in the salivary glands.

This scenario of unintentional receptor binding and thus unanticipated side effects is quite common, but luckily, not all of the effects will occur at the same drug dose. To prevent the occurrence of many undesired effects, drugs are typically designed to produce their therapeutic (desired) effect at low concentrations, so that they are less likely to produce strong effects from unintentional binding to other receptors. Consequently, although the desired and undesired effects both occur because of drug-receptor interaction, you are more likely to experience side effects when you take higher doses of your medications.

PREDICTING DRUG EFFECTS IN AN INDIVIDUAL

We have now learned about the processes of drug binding and activation or blocking of receptors in the body (pharmacodynamics). We also understand the processes by which drugs reach their site(s) of action (pharmacokinetics). Does that mean than we can reliably predict what a certain dose of a drug will do in a certain person? The answer is that we can do it to some extent, but there are several points to be considered:

1. Factors such as age, weight, and genetics may affect the absorption, distribution, metabolism, and excretion processes and therefore change an individual's response to a drug, as outlined in Chapter 3.
2. Since most drugs enhance or block the activity of endogenous substances, their effect may depend on how much endogenous substance you produce, and this may also differ among individuals.
3. Beyond the genetic variability of metabolizing enzymes as we discussed in the case of CYP enzymes in Chapter 3, there is a genetic variability in drug receptors so that one person may have more, or less, of these receptors available, or have a slightly different receptor structure that will affect how well a certain drug will bind to it.

There are drugs for which known parameters can affect their desired and undesired effects, and your physician will consider parameters such as your weight or age before deciding on the dose of the medication to prescribe. For other drugs, laboratory tests such as kidney and liver function can further guide the decision for selecting more appropriate doses. In addition, there is a subset of drugs (mostly used for cancer treatment and for preventing blood clots), for which your doctor may order genetic testing to further guide treatment. In many other cases, because known predictive parameters are lacking, the dose is selected by "titration to response," which means that you will be initially prescribed a low dose of a drug and your doctor will monitor its desired and undesired effects and, based on these, will determine whether further dose increase is necessary. Sometimes, multiple dose-modification steps will be necessary to find the dose that achieves its desired outcomes but does not cause side effects.

THE PLACEBO EFFECT

In pharmacodynamics, there is an important component that is often overlooked, or even ignored. I mentioned earlier that the presence and the amount of the endogenous substances may affect the drug effects. Since our body is the one producing these endogenous molecules, it is important to understand that our emotional state, our beliefs, and our expectations can seriously influence the effects of treatment. I will even take it a step further and say that in some circumstances, the extent of our emotions, beliefs, and expectations may make as much difference as the full effect of a drug we take.

I mentioned in Chapter 2 that to find whether a drug is truly effective, it usually needs to be compared to an inactive substance, a *placebo*. One of the reasons is that if you think that you are taking a fantastic drug and it is going to cure you, the chances that this happens are actually in your favor. This phenomenon, which is attributed to the psychological effect of taking the drug, or the expectation of it, is called *the placebo response*. The word "placebo" originates from Latin *placēbō*, and its source has been attributed as a reference to "fake" mourners—people who would come to a funeral, falsely claiming a connection with the deceased, to get food and drink. Accordingly, *placebo* has often been treated as a bad or negative manipulation. But in the context of medical treatment, especially when it's your own treatment, I strongly disagree that the placebo response is "cheating." If a certain effect can be achieved by expectation or anticipation, then both the patient and the caregiver benefit from it. If taking one analgesic pill and believing it will work does the same job as taking three pills but not believing they will work, then the former option is definitely preferable.

What I am saying is that drugs often enhance or inhibit activities that occur in our body anyway. If you can find a way of enhancing or inhibiting the activity of certain hormones and neurotransmitters by the power of thought, anticipation, excitation, breathing, or yoga—why wouldn't you? Think about it. We can sometimes be in the middle of some activity (ball game, running, playing, fighting) and hurt ourselves and not even notice we did. When we discover the cut after the activity we wonder how it could have gone unnoticed. If that injury had occurred in a quiet room, it would certainly have hurt. That means that our body has certain ability to provide a painkiller effect by itself, and harnessing that ability for our own benefit is not a bad thing.

Importantly, placebo effect is more likely to influence measures that are subjectively experienced by a person rather than those measured by objective tests. Beliefs and expectations are more likely to influence symptoms related to pain, depression, anxiety, and poor sleep quality than affect results of blood tests, x-ray scans, or blood pressure measures taken in the physician's office. With that said, a study published in the *New England Journal of Medicine* had shown that the symptoms of some people with Parkinson's disease, which is a severe neurological disorder, improved after a *sham* brain surgery, likely by the virtue of belief that they were transplanted special cells in the brain that would produce the deficient neurotransmitter *dopamine*.

The rationale for highlighting the placebo effect in this chapter is that while drugs are developed in the laboratory to act on certain receptor targets to produce known and specific pharmacodynamic effects, several factors such as your expectations and emotional state, which are beyond the prescribing physician's control, can influence how you would respond to a drug. Therefore, it is important to keep in mind the effect that placebo can have on our daily medication intake and its results.

Take-Home Message

Drugs are typically designed to act on receptors to hormones, neurotransmitters, and growth factors—which are molecules produced by our own body. By either acting as agonists (activators) or antagonists (blockers) of these receptors, most drugs attempt to correct the imbalance or the underlying pathology created by a disease or a condition. The knowledge of how your drugs engage with their biological targets can assist in understanding and appropriately addressing the desired and undesired effects of your drugs. Importantly, your state of mind, beliefs, and expectations can change the balance of hormones and neurotransmitters in your body and thus change your response to certain drugs.

[5]

TAKING MY DRUGS PROPERLY

Most of us wish to live longer but also to have decent quality of life that enables us to do things that make us happy and our lives more interesting. That's easy enough if you are healthy, but for the 45% of the population who have at least one chronic disease that negatively affects life expectancy or quality, it's not that simple. Many diseases and conditions have genetic, age-related, environmental, or other causes that we are currently unable to prevent. Fortunately, for our generation, though, modern medicine has decent tools to deal with most chronic conditions. It is true that some diseases are more challenging to treat than others, but for many, achieving reasonable therapy goals is certainly possible, and doing so can allow reasonable life expectancy and quality of life. Lifestyle changes, diet, psychological therapy, surgery, radiation, acupuncture, and many other approaches can be used for treating diseases, but since this book will focus on pharmacological approaches, I am obviously going to discuss how to maximize the benefits and minimize the risks of drugs.

ADHERENCE TO TREATMENT

It is correct to assume that a drug that was approved for marketing by authorities such as the US Food and Drug Administration (FDA) and European Medicines Agency (EMA) should be safe (enough) and effective (enough). Indeed, pharmaceutical companies spend 10 to 12 years researching the effectiveness and safety of each drug, the results of which are meticulously reviewed by the regulatory authorities before approving the drug to be marketed. There is a catch, though: the medications will usually work, and do so safely, *only* if taken *properly* for the *appropriate* conditions. In fact, lack of adherence to a treatment regimen is one of the major reasons for therapy failure in many diseases, such as epilepsy, asthma, bacterial infections, and HIV. *Adherence* means *sticking to* your prescribed drug regimen, or faithfully taking the drugs as prescribed.

When medications are prescribed, the usual expectation is that you are going to adhere to the prescribed regimen. Unfortunately, the statistics on adherence do not look good. The World Health Organization (WHO) reported that adherence rates to drug therapy in chronic conditions average only 50% in developed countries. As an example, a study of more than 700,000 patients compared adherence rates among six chronic diseases and looked at only one component of adherence—patients who over 1 year obtained at least 80% of the medication supply from the pharmacy (these patients were considered to have good adherence). The best adherence rates were among patients with high blood pressure—but still only 72% of them obtained their medications. Among patients with seizure disorders, only 61%, and among patients with osteoporosis, only 51% obtained their medications. And this study did not even assess whether the patients had been taking their medicines properly, which is another big nonadherence component. So the physicians may prescribe the most appropriate medications, but if only 50 to 60% of the people obtain the drugs that were prescribed, you probably agree that we are facing some serious barriers for appropriately treating chronic conditions.

WHY IS IT SO DIFFICULT TO ADHERE TO A MEDICATION REGIMEN?

Doesn't it seem rational that people who have a disease and want it treated or cured will adhere to their treatment? Who wouldn't want their condition to be well managed? Well, it appears that rationale and logic are not the only contributors to good adherence. Dan Ariely, a professor of psychology and behavioral economics, elegantly describes this conundrum in his book called *The Upside of Irrationality: Unexpected Benefits of Defying Logic.* He highlights our tendency as humans to overemphasize the present over the long-term, whether related to decisions about exercise, diet, or finances. As a result, even though it makes complete sense to remember to take your daily medications to prevent something major like liver failure or heart attack, most people will have difficulty with daily adherence without any sort of immediate reward, particularly if the drugs cause unpleasant side effects.

In my experience, another big challenge for patients, when they are diagnosed with a new condition or prescribed a new drug, is the *adaptation to change.* Change is hard for almost anyone, and we all know how difficult it is to change routines. One of the most striking cases of a rapid and unexpected change occurs in people who have a heart attack (*acute myocardial infarction*) for the first time. Many of these individuals are middle-aged men who have considered themselves relatively healthy. Well, maybe a bit overweight, smoking, and not very active physically, but they might not have considered these as serious health issues, or at least serious enough to warrant engaging in routine exercise and weight loss programs. And one day, out of the blue, they have a heart attack. If they survive it, the standard drug regimen for preventing the second heart attack is quite a massive package, and typically includes the following:

1. A once- or twice-a-day pill called an *ACE inhibitor* (see Chapter 11) that prevents further damage to the heart muscle and reduces blood pressure, if necessary;

2. A drug called a *beta-blocker* (see Chapter 11) that, by reducing heart rate and oxygen requirements of the heart, helps prevent future heart attacks;

3. A once-a-day pill for lowering cholesterol (called a *statin*; see Chapter 12) that will be prescribed even if cholesterol levels are not very high; and

4. A once-a-day aspirin pill, and perhaps an additional blood thinner (see Chapter 13).

Imagine—within a 48 hours, you go from zero pills a day to taking four to six pills a day to maximize your chances of preventing another, potentially fatal, heart attack. And all this might not be sufficient—you will also need to get more physically active, lose some weight, and quit smoking to improve your chances of survival.

Can a person make all these lifestyle changes and, on top of that, add several daily medications that may cause some side effects? Well, it is going to be difficult. I will say it again. **IT IS GOING TO BE DIFFICULT**. But honestly, there might be no other way around it. Quoting Albert Einstein: "it is foolish to do the same thing again and again and expect a different outcome." If you don't want a second heart attack, which could kill you, you don't have much choice but to get used to this new life of yours—which could actually be of similar quality and duration as anyone else's if you achieve the desired treatment goals. And the good news is: **IT IS POSSIBLE**. It's not going to work for everyone, but with the right amount of guidance from healthcare professionals and the right amount of responsibility on your behalf, the majority of contributing factors can be reasonably managed to prevent the next heart attack. And this approach is true for many other long-term conditions.

But remember: no one can force you to take this responsibility. **It is going to be your own choice as an individual either to decide to live a longer and healthier life and get the maximum from the only life you get, or to decide that it is too much to bother, take your medications whenever you remember to do so, leave your health to chance, and hope for a miracle.**

So what stands between "**it is possible**" and actually making your treatment work? Despite a variety of factors that can affect treatment success, I believe there are three key components to successful drug therapy, and they can be formulated as three simple questions. If you have been properly educated about the right answers to all three questions for each of your medications, and you actually act on the last two, my experience shows that your chances of achieving the treatment goals are going to increase tremendously. These questions are:

1. *Why* should I take my medication?
2. *How* should I take my medication?
3. *What* should I measure to track the treatment success?

The answers to each of these three questions are going to be unique to you because probably no one else has exactly the same set of circumstances as you do. The rest of the chapter is going to discuss these three questions, their importance, and what they consist of. This book as a whole is intended to provide you with sufficient fundamental knowledge for understanding these components. Based on what is relevant to you, you can then help your physician construct the optimal treatment plan for you, one that you can make work to achieve your treatment goals. And if you find ways to reward yourself for achieving weekly treatment goals, you can improve your treatment success even further.

QUESTION 1: *WHY* SHOULD I TAKE MY MEDICATION?

Any behavioral psychologist, fitness coach, or life coach will tell you that a key requirement for achieving a goal is attaching a **purpose** to that goal. When you have a *clearly outlined purpose*—whether for losing weight, reaching a certain financial or career target, or any other goal in life—it subconsciously supports the continuous effort you need to put in to reach that goal. It is not different with your health and medications. A key requirement is understanding WHY you should take these drugs—*what is the purpose?* To fulfill that requirement, you need to understand the condition you are suffering from and its implications on your life. Some conditions may be simply a nuisance—and although you have them, after learning about them and discussing them with your physician, you may decide that you don't want them to be treated. That is absolutely fine. Your body—your decision. Other conditions, if untreated, may substantially impair your quality of life or increase the risk for disability or death. When you clearly understand the short-term and long-term consequences of not treating your condition—then the purpose, or the answer to the WHY question, becomes very clear. This is when you understand what you've got to lose if you don't achieve your treatment goal. And again, it is going to be *your* choice. Unless you *believe* that treating a certain disease is important for *you*, you are not very likely to adhere to your treatment and achieve your treatment goals. This is clear beyond any doubt. Get the information, discuss with your healthcare professional, and if you are not going to treat the condition, don't bother and don't waste time and resources. My only advice is that you make sure that you CLEARLY understand the risks and the benefits of not treating a certain condition, specific details of which will be outlined in Chapters 11 to 20.

After you understand the disease and you are prescribed a drug (or few drugs) to treat it, the need for reliable information on how much the prescribed treatment is expected to improve your condition is key. Not every treatment may be worth its side effects. But when you understand the expected benefit to your health and consider the potential risks, you will then get a reliable answer to the question: *Why* should I take my medications? It is one thing to be told that you have diabetes and you need to take these three drugs and lose weight, and it's another thing to understand that untreated diabetes substantially increases your risk for blindness, kidney failure, chronic pain, amputation of your legs, and the likelihood of dying early from a heart attack or a stroke, and that achieving your diabetes treatment goals with medications and lifestyle changes is actually going to reduce these risks.

Matching a Drug to a Disease

When clinical pharmacy specialists perform medication therapy evaluation (also called a comprehensive drug review), one of the first things they assess is whether each disease is properly managed and whether all the drugs the patient takes have clear indications (i.e., reasons for taking). This schematically may look like the following list:

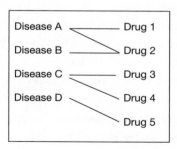

I encourage every person who takes medications to make such a list for themselves. In a discussion with your physician, it should be decided which conditions should be treated with medications. As I mentioned, some may not need treatment at all. Then, based on the treatment goals, each disease that requires drug therapy should be treated with the optimal medication or combination of medications. In parallel, it is important to make sure that each drug you take is treating a certain condition. I often see patients who were prescribed a drug years ago and keep taking it without even remembering what the drugs is for and without knowing what benefit to expect from it. Each drug may cause side effects, and the larger the quantity of your daily medications, the bigger the risk for side effects and undesired interactions between the drugs. You should only take drugs that are prescribed with a clear purpose of treating your conditions. Your pharmacist can be a great resource to help out in this process.

The "why should I take my medication" question is relevant for even the simplest of treatments—a 10-day antibiotic course for a sore throat. This sort of treatment regimen typically includes taking a capsule twice a day (a total of 20 doses); however, a huge amount of people will fill the prescription late or won't take the 20 doses as prescribed. Some will miss a few doses simply because they forgot or were busy, some will experience certain side effects and therefore skip doses, and others will feel better after 3 days and decide they had enough antibiotics and stop the treatment. This could happen without, or despite, clear directions from the physician that in order for the treatment to succeed, and to prevent complications, the antibiotic needs to be taken twice a day for the full 10 days.

Whether the instructions were provided or not, it is your responsibility, as a patient, to clearly understand the treatment goals and the risks of not treating the infection properly. "Killing the bacteria" is not a good enough goal for treating a sore throat because it is not a tangible concept, and it is not the *real* goal. The true *purpose* of a full 10-day antibiotic treatment is relieving your fever and associated symptoms, decreasing the duration of the illness, limiting household spread of the infection, preventing the bacteria from developing resistance to the antibiotic, and preventing rheumatic fever—a condition resulting from inadequately treated sore throat that can cause permanent damage to your heart.

Bottom line: get your physician's help in defining the true purpose of treating your condition—that is, *why* you should take your medications. It will make a big change in the way you perceive the treatment.

QUESTION 2: *HOW* SHOULD I TAKE MY MEDICATIONS?

After it has been decided that condition X requires treatment with medication and the *why* question is answered, the next step is to understand *how* to take the drugs optimally to achieve the treatment goals. This is a question to which many of the details throughout this book become handy because the answer may be complex at times. The answer will require processing of different types of information, such as drug pharmacokinetics and pharmacodynamics that we discussed earlier, and knowledge on drug interactions and undesired effects that I will discuss in the subsequent chapters.

Wouldn't it be ideal if all the drugs you needed were small and tasty, could be taken by mouth once a day (or, even better, once a month), all at the same time, and would provide full benefit? It probably would, but modern medicine is not there yet. Based on parameters such as the extent of a drug's absorption to the bloodstream (i.e., bioavailability) and the speed at which the drug is excreted from the body (i.e., drug's *half-life*—as mentioned in Chapter 3), it is often impossible to administer a drug once a day and sometimes is not even possible to take it by mouth. Drugs with a short half-life may need to be taken every few hours, and drugs that are poorly absorbed from the gastrointestinal tract won't even be available as pills but only as injections or inhalers. For these reasons, some drugs should be taken 3 times a day, others as a pill once a week, and some applied as a patch on the skin every 72 hours. For someone who takes several drugs with variable administration regimens, proper adherence often becomes a real challenge, hindering the ability to achieve optimal treatment outcomes.

These challenges certainly exist, but there are also practical solutions to many of them. Without going too much into the specifics, I will outline in this section what could the different considerations be properly taking your medications, some potential pitfalls, and tips that could help you make sure that the *how* question is answered properly and that you are indeed taking your drugs as intended.

A basic requirement is to understand what your drug label consists of in order to avoid misinterpretation and subsequent medication errors. Figure 5.1 illustrates an example of a drug label that could appear on a bottle of *diphenhydramine* your physician prescribed for the treatment of your allergy symptoms. The sections that follow, along with general guidance on *how* to take your medication, will provide more detailed description of the different components of the drug label.

1. Drug's Generic Name versus Trade Name

The *generic name* is the name of the actual active molecule of the drug. It refers to its chemical composition and not to a manufacturer or advertisement. When you take a pill, it contains the active component and a variety of other components (called *excipients*) that give the pill its shape, color, taste, and size and that hold the active component together. Each drug has one (or sometimes

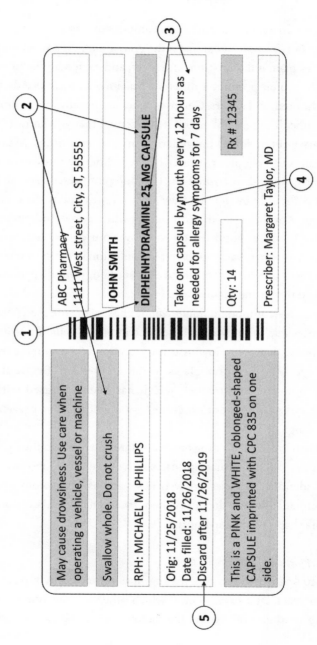

May cause drowsiness. Use care when operating a vehicle, vessel or machine

Swallow whole. Do not crush

RPH: MICHAEL M. PHILLIPS

Orig: 11/25/2018
Date filled: 11/26/2018
Discard after 11/26/2019

This is a PINK and WHITE, oblonged-shaped CAPSULE imprinted with CPC 835 on one side.

ABC Pharmaey
1111 West street, City, ST, 55555

JOHN SMITH

DIPHENHYDRAMINE 25 MG CAPSULE

Take one capsule by mouth every 12 hours as needed for allergy symptoms for 7 days

Qty: 14   Rx # 12345

Prescriber: Margaret Taylor, MD

Figure 5.1. Example of a drug label. The *circled numbers* correspond to the number of the section in which the relevant information appears in the chapter.

more) active components, and each component has a unique *generic name*. For example, *ibuprofen* is the *generic name* of a substance that reduces pain, inflammation, and fever, and each manufacturer gives its ibuprofen product a different *trade name*, such as Advil, Motrin, Nurofen, and others. Generic names are usually more complex and difficult to remember, but it is essential that you know (or at least have written down) the generic names of your drugs. Many errors occur when people are prescribed two different trade names of the same generic drug (usually by two different prescribers) and take both without knowing that they are merely doubling the dose of one drug. Another type of error occurs when two brand names sound alike (another good reason to know your generic names). The FDA often issues warnings to avoid confusion in drugs' names, based on cases in which people were prescribed, were dispensed, or had taken the wrong medication. For example, the eye medicine **Durezol** (active component *difluprednate*) has been confused with a wart remover solution **Durasal** (active component *salicylic acid*), resulting in eye damage following the application of a wart remover into the eye. Another example is an antidepressant **Brintellix** (active component *vortioxetine*), which has been confused with **Brilinta** (active component *ticagrelor*)—a medication to prevent blood clotting.

If you have misplaced a drug or are not sure you received the right drug, you can call a pharmacy or use some of the online resources (e.g., pill identifier features on websites such as Drugs.com and RxList.com) and identify the pill's generic/brand name and the dose by the pill's shape, color, and imprint.

Approval of Generic Drug Products
When a company markets a new drug, it is protected by a patent for several years, after expiration of which other manufacturers are allowed to produce and market that active compound as a *generic*

drug. Two *generic drugs* will have the same active component at the same dose. The FDA approves generic drugs based on their chemical composition, physical properties, and research in healthy volunteers demonstrating that taking the two drugs does not result in significant difference in pharmacokinetics (parameters such as bioavailability and maximum blood concentration; see Chapter 3). Generic drugs and the original drug are interchangeable, so for the same prescription you may sometimes get a drug with one trade name and sometimes with another. For the vast majority of patients, both drugs will result in the same effect. However, two generic products do not necessarily have the same excipients, or the same size and taste of the product. In rare cases, people may have allergies to *excipients* that are present in one drug product but not in the other or have difficulty with swallowing a certain drug because of its size, shape, or taste. Some people report differences in effectiveness or side effects, which are sometimes perceived (because they believe or expect one drug to work better) and sometimes real, especially with certain drugs for treating asthma or seizures, which I will discuss in Chapters 15 and 16.

2. Drug's Formulation

Formulation is the final composition of a medicinal product. For example, the *acetaminophen* (generic name) product called Tylenol (trade name) can be marketed in various *formulations,* such as Tylenol tablets, Tylenol oral liquid, and Tylenol 8-hour extended-release tablets. All these formulations of *acetaminophen* are to be taken by mouth, but they may differ in regard to certain characteristics, such as their *onset* and *duration* of action or the suitability of administration in children.

The most common *oral liquid* formulations of drugs include *syrups,* which usually have a certain amount of sugar that helps stabilize the drug and mask unpleasant tastes that some drugs have, *oral solutions* in which usually a water-soluble drug is dissolved in the liquid, and *suspensions* in which drug particles float in the liquid—and these will usually require shaking the bottle before drug administration, like many antibiotic oral liquid formulations. The liquid formulations are more suitable for children who have difficulty swallowing pills or individuals who need fine adjustment of drug doses because it's easier to control the amount of intake for a liquid drug.

Oral solid formulations may differ significantly as well because they can appear as tablets or capsules of various sizes and shapes. Most oral solid formulations are designed as *immediate release* drugs, which means that the pill is broken down and releases the active drug in its entirety when it reaches the stomach. Some drugs are *enteric coated*, which means they will release their contents rapidly, but it will happen only after the drug leaves the stomach and moves to the small intestine because the pill is coated by a film that is resistant to the acidic environment of the stomach. This technique is usually reserved for drugs that irritate the stomach when taken by mouth—for example, aspirin.

Other oral drugs have formulations that allow *modified release* and can have several possible *titles* such as *controlled release, sustained release,* and *extended release.* These differ from each other but generally are intended to allow the active drug to be released from the pill at a slower rate, which can serve several purposes. If the drug itself is short-acting and requires several daily doses, an extended-release formulation will allow taking a larger dose of the drug, but a dose that is slowly released in the intestines over several hours, which will allow once-a-day or twice-a-day administration. This can be a great advantage in terms of convenience. On the other hand, it may mean that the total dose of the drug "loaded" into the pill is higher, and if you chew the pill (instead of swallowing it) the structure that allows the modified release will be damaged, and higher pill contents will be released immediately and cause undesired effects. So as a rule, modified-release pills are to be swallowed whole.

Ask your doctor or pharmacist about your prescribed drug's formulation. Understanding the release, onset, and duration properties of your drug will help you navigate better toward its beneficial and safe use.

3. Drugs' Dose and Frequency

Very often, the drug's dose will determine its effectiveness and also its undesired effects. The most common units of drug dose are expressed in **milligrams** (**mg**). The drug's label will always carry the information of the drug's *generic name* and its *dose* (in other words, strength). For example, in the drug label shown in Figure 5.1, each capsule contains 25 mg of the active component *diphenhydramine*.

For some substances, other dose units are acceptable—for example, *vitamin D* dose will be expressed in units—such as 1000 international units (IU) per capsule. Liquid drugs will frequently bear a *concentration* label—that is, amount of the drug in a certain volume of the liquid. For example—an antibiotic suspension may read "250 mg of *amoxicillin* per 5 mL of suspension" (or "*amoxicillin*, 250 mg in 5 mL"). That means that each teaspoon (5 mL) of the ready and shaken suspension contains 250 mg of the drug, and if the doctor has prescribed you a 10-mL dose 3 times a day, you will receive 500 mg of *amoxicillin* 3 times a day.

Insulin product doses will appear in units of injectable solution. Your prescription may be for a certain type of *insulin* at a dose of 25 units twice a day before meals. A syringe does not inject units but rather a certain volume of a solution. Therefore, you should read the label, which will say that there are "100 units of *insulin* per each mL solution," and you need to obtain a certain syringe or injection pen that can help you convert the required *dose* (i.e., 25 units) to eventual *volume* (i.e., one fourth of a milliliter—0.25 mL) of the solution that will be injected.

The drug dose will be decided by your physician based on several factors. Some drugs have standard doses; for other drugs, your individual dose may be determined based on your weight, age, condition, liver and kidney function, and sometimes other laboratory test results. It is important to clearly understand what is the *daily* dose that you need to take versus the dose per each administration (e.g., of a pill, a syrup, an injection) and the *frequency* of administration. With once-daily dosing, the single dose will also be the daily dose, but as I mentioned, many drugs cannot be administered once a day. For example, if you are prescribed *gabapentin* with a dose of 600 mg every 8 hours for treating pain after nerve damage, the single dose is 600 mg (which might be taken as two capsules of 300-mg strength each), and your daily dose is 1800 mg.

Timing is also important, even with once-a-day drugs. Some drugs may cause drowsiness and might be better taken before sleep to prevent symptoms during the day. Other drugs may increase alertness and are better taken in the morning so that they do not interfere with sleep. As I will discuss in later chapters, drugs for treating high cholesterol, for example, are usually taken in the evening because the liver is producing most of the cholesterol at night, so you want to "target" peak cholesterol production with high concentration of the drug.

If the drug is intended to be taken several times a day, it is important to clarify the optimal time for taking the drug. For twice-a-day dosing, roughly every 12 hours (e.g., 8 a.m. and 8 p.m. or 9 p.m.) should work well for most drugs. If you are prescribed a 3-times-a-day drug (and you sleep 9 hours at night), you typically don't need to wake up to take a drug exactly every 8 hours—a 9-hour interval should be fine for most drugs. Some drugs, however, may require *asymmetric* dosing. For example, *nitrate* drugs for treating heart conditions might need to be taken with a 7- to 8-hour interval, then allowing the body a 16- to 17-hour nitrate-free period to recover.

To summarize: it is important to understand what dose of the drug you are prescribed, what constitutes each dose (e.g., two pills, 5 mL of syrup, two puffs of asthma inhaler), and what the frequency of administration is. Depending on your drug, your condition, and your typical daily activities, be sure to consult your physician or pharmacist on how to plan the dosing schedule optimally through the day.

4. Drug's Route of Administration

Route of administration is basically the pathway by which the drug enters the body. The correct route is also of critical importance. Although the majority of drugs are administered by mouth to be swallowed, there exist a variety of other possible administration routes. Intravenous (IV) injection is one common route, although it typically requires a hospital or clinic setting and medical personnel to administer the drug. IV injections are intended for fast and complete delivery of the drug to the bloodstream, avoiding absorption issues and the lag time required for absorption. Other types of injections such as *subcutaneous* (under the skin) are becoming more common, especially with biological drugs such as proteins and antibodies, and many patients are increasingly using this route of administration at home. There are more sophisticated ways of delivering drugs to the site of their action to achieve high local concentration and minimize *systemic* spread, for example, injection into the joints (*intra-articular*) or close to the spinal nerves and spinal cord (*epidural* or *intrathecal*), but these are performed by trained healthcare professionals.

Another route of administration involves drugs used at home that may require direct delivery to the airway by inhalation to treat airway or lung diseases (discussed more thoroughly in Chapter 15). Other drugs are better and faster absorbed from the small blood vessels inside the mouth and under the tongue than from the stomach. This method of administration for direct absorption from the oral cavity (termed *sublingual,* or *buccal*), circumventing the stomach, is common for *vitamin B₁₂,* some analgesics for severe pain, and *nitro-glycerin* for heart conditions. Nasal sprays can be used to treat local conditions or actually deliver drugs to the nasal cavity for systemic absorption, similarly to the sublingual methods.

Delivery to the skin in creams, ointments, and patches can be used for treating local (*topical*) skin conditions. On the other hand, skin can be used for delivery of drugs to the bloodstream because some drugs are poorly absorbed from the intestine but have certain properties that allow them to penetrate the skin and reach the blood vessels in the deeper layers of the skin. This route of administration is called *transdermal*—that is, crossing the skin. Transdermal patches are often used for treating pain, but it is important to understand that as opposed to local treatments that should be applied at the painful area, the area of transdermal patch application has nothing to do with the painful area. The shoulders and upper back are the more appropriate areas for trans-dermal patch applications; the drug is supposed to be absorbed to the systemic circulation and reach its site of action through the bloodstream.

Drugs can be also delivered rectally, vaginally, and sometimes in more invasive methods to cavities such as the bladder or the uterus—for treating local disorders or for systemic delivery. While working in a community pharmacy, I have encountered patients who have swallowed their rectal suppositories, used vaginal suppositories rectally, used eye drops orally—and in most of the cases, it has been a lack of proper instruction by the healthcare team, coupled with not reading the drug label and instructions. None of these interventions worked, of course, and these all were easily preventable errors.

To summarize: administering the right drug at the right dose by the *wrong* route is usually not going to work and, in some cases, may cause damage. Therefore, it is important to clearly understand by which route the drug is to be taken.

The drug label will typically include an accurate description of how to take it. If you need additional information, you can consult your pharmacist or use an online resource such as the WHO's *Guide to Good Prescribing*, which contains detailed explanations on how to correctly use drugs for various routes, such as eye drops, transdermal patches, suppositories, and others.

5. Drug's Expiration and Storage

Each drug has an expiration date beyond which it is no longer approved to be used. It will be stamped on the original manufacturer's package or on the pharmacy label attached to the drug container (see Figure 5.1). If only the month and the year are indicated, the expiration date refers to the *last* day of that month.

There are several reasons drugs have expiration dates. More commonly, the drug composition is affected after a certain period of time—the contact with air (or water for liquid drugs) may cause oxidation or breakdown of the drug, and the amount of the active component will be lower than initially prescribed. The regulatory agencies allow for about 10% variation in active drug over the product's "shelf-life" and typically give 2 to 5 years from manufacturing until expiration to most drugs, based on stability tests provided by the manufacturer. Sometimes the decision is based on sterility issues or other consideration that affect a drug's composition and dose. Uncommonly, drugs are broken down over time to form toxic compounds, and the use of such drugs beyond their expiration date may not be safe. The reality is that probably about 60 to 70% of drugs in oral solid dosage forms (e.g., tablets and capsules) still retain close to 100% of their initial composition even 1 to 2 years after their formal expiration date. However, because the information on what happens with each individual drug beyond its expiration is not available, given the concerns with safety and effectiveness with some drugs, simply *do not use drugs beyond their expiration date*—in particular drugs for injection or those in nonsolid formulations.

The expiration date also depends on storage conditions: it attests to the stability of the drug if stored in proper condition as indicated on the label, which is typically in a cool and dry place, without exposure to heat and moisture. If the drugs were exposed to extreme conditions (e.g., left inside the car for many hours in hot weather), consult with your pharmacist or the drug manufacturer about how the conditions may have affected stability and the expiration date. The manufacturers often have some stability data to provide more reliable answers regarding continued use. As a rule of thumb, if your medicine looks different (i.e., changed color, looks "old,") or smells different, do not take it. Note that liquid dosage forms and biological products, like insulin or other injectable proteins, are more sensitive to suboptimal storage conditions and often require refrigeration.

In general, heat, light, air, and moisture can damage drugs. Although many people store their drugs in a medicine cabinet in their bathroom, it is actually not a good practice because the bathroom is usually hotter and moister than other rooms. A dresser drawer or storage box in a closet or the kitchen, as long as it is stored well away from hot appliances, would be a safer option than the so-called medicine cabinet in your bathroom.

After understanding the five previous sections as they pertain to the instructions on the drug label, you should also inquire about your drug's relevance to food, beverages, and other drugs you are taking. These details are important to the effectiveness and the safety of your drugs and will be discussed in detail in Chapter 6.

It may be difficult to remember all those details pertaining to all your drugs. Fortunately, there are excellent smartphone applications available (Round Health, Pill and Med Reminder, Pill Reminder, and others at the time of writing), which allow you to enter all the information about each of your drug's name, dose, route, and frequency so that (1) you have the current list of medications that you easily update every time you start, stop, or change a drug; and (2) you can set reminders/alarms to take your medications on time.

To summarize: the question of *how* to take the medication may seem trivial, but previously outlined components are all important and can affect your treatment, especially if the treatment regimen is complex. These considerations are of particular importance when decisions need be made regarding a switch to a generic drug or a different formulation, a change in dosing regimen, or drug exposure to suboptimal storing conditions.

QUESTION 3: *WHAT* SHOULD I MEASURE TO TRACK THE TREATMENT SUCCESS?

I will repeat a part of the sentence I mentioned in question 1 earlier: "understanding that untreated diabetes substantially increases your risk for blindness . . . or a stroke; and that achieving your diabetes treatment goals with medications . . . is actually going to reduce these risks." Note, that I did not write that "taking your medications is actually going to reduce these risks," but rather, "**achieving your diabetes treatment goals** with medications and lifestyle changes is actually going to reduce these risks."

Lord Kelvin (1824–1907), best known for his work on determining the absolute zero temperature and developing the Kelvin temperature scale, is the source of one of my most favorite quotes: "If you cannot measure it, you cannot improve it." Knowledge about your condition (question 1) and adherence to the prescribed treatment (question 2) are a great step forward but may not suffice to ensure you are properly treated. There is more to successful treatment than prescribing an appropriate drug for a condition. This third, crucial component is to define *what* the desired treatment outcomes are and *what* to measure to determine success. This element is probably the trickiest among the three and requires the most active day-to-day involvement on your part.

The choice of "what to measure as success" substantially varies from condition to condition and from person to person. For example, if you have high blood pressure, important measurements of success could be the prevention of complications such as a heart attack and stroke over the next 20 years. But the occurrence of a stroke or a heart attack is not a continuous measure; we cannot monitor it daily because it is a discrete event that will either occur or not within that 20-year time frame we defined. And when either a stroke or heart attack occurs, it's too late. But research shows that actually by controlling the blood pressure, these complications of the disease can be prevented. For many conditions in which the desired outcome cannot be monitored directly, we have "surrogate" measures, which are readily available measures that give a good approximation of the true outcome we are trying to achieve.

Therefore, if you have high blood pressure and are prescribed drugs for it, your physician will set a goal for blood pressure (e.g., below 130/85 mm Hg), and although it may not always be easily achieved, the goal is clear and the measurement of blood pressure at home is quite straightforward.

In other conditions, such as chronic pain, the outcomes might be neither easily measurable nor clear. If you report chronic low back pain with average pain intensity of 6 on a 0 to 10 scale, the goal may be set for reducing this pain, for example, to 3 on a 0 to 10 scale. However, the appropriateness of this outcomes measure can be argued, considering that the decrease in pain intensity per se does not necessarily mean that you have gained additional quality of life or have functionally improved. It would be necessary to assess your functional status to obtain a measurable outcome that is **important to you**. In this case, if your pain intensity is reduced to 4, but you are sleeping better, are able to work a full day, and are able to spend more time with friends and family, the treatment may be considered successful, as opposed to a situation in which the pain is reduced to 3, but you have not improved on those measures of function and quality of life. Unfortunately, there is no single formula here—for one person the desired outcome would be the ability to go back to work, and for another person the functional outcome would be improving the emotional aspect of anxiety associated with pain. For subjectively assessed conditions such as pain and depression, it would be important to set up treatment goals that are important to **you** and to decide what individual measures should be tracked for successful treatment.

After we have discussed the previous three questions, let's take an example of two individuals and look at the differences in formulating their treatment plans.

Linda is a 67-year-old woman with high cholesterol levels and high blood pressure who is mildly overweight. She is retired, enjoys gardening, is active in the community, and helps her daughter with grandchildren care.

Michael is a 52-year-old moderately overweight man with diabetes and low back pain. He is married and has three children. Michael works part-time as a software engineer; back pain limits work for more than 3 consecutive hours a day. He is struggling to support his family because he is unable to work full-time.

There is a variety of ways to formulate individual plans for Linda and Michael, and the way the plan is formulated can affect the success of the treatment.

For Linda, the plan could be as follows (but in no way should the specific drugs be taken as relevant to you, the reader—consult your physician first):

- Take *simvastatin* 20 mg once a day to reduce blood levels of cholesterol.
- Take *ramipril* 5 mg once a day and *atenolol* 50 mg once a day to reduce blood pressure.
- Lose weight.

For Michael, the plan could look as follows (but again, in no way should this be taken as relevant to you, the reader):

- Take *metformin* 850 mg 3 times a day and *glyburide* 5 mg twice a day to control diabetes.
- Take *acetaminophen* 1000 mg 3 times a day and *gabapentin* 600 mg 3 times a day to reduce pain.
- Lose weight by diet and exercise.

Alternatively, these plans could be based on the three-step plan as discussed in this chapter and outlined in a table form like in Table 5.1.

TABLE 5.1 AN OUTLINE FOR A THREE-STEP (*WHY/HOW/WHAT*) PLAN FOR MEDICATIONS

Condition	1. *Why* Treat?	2. Medications and *How* to Take Them	3. *What* to Measure	Desired Outcome
A		1		
		2		
B		1		
		2		

You can draw this sort of a table for yourself on a paper using a pencil or create it in a computer spreadsheet, whichever works best for you.

Detailed outlines of contents for such a table for Linda and Michael are provided here.

A *Why/How/What* Plan for **Linda's** Medications

I. **High cholesterol**

1. *Why treat?*

Increases the chance of heart disease and early disability or death from heart attack or stroke. Won't be able to continue gardening, community activities, and spending time with grandchildren.

2. *Medications and how to take them*

Simvastatin 20-mg pill. Take by mouth once a day at 7 p.m., after dinner.

3. *What to measure*

Blood tests every 3 months to measure LDL (low-density lipoprotein) and total cholesterol

Desired outcome

LDL below 129 mg/dL

II. High blood pressure

1. *Why treat?*

Same as for high cholesterol

2. *Medications and how to take them*

Ramipril 5-mg pill. Take by mouth once a day at 8 a.m.

Atenolol 50-mg pill. Take by mouth once a day at 8 a.m.

3. *What to measure*

Daily home measurement of blood pressure while sitting. Keep diary of the measurements. Bring for primary care physician (PCP) assessment every 3 months.

Desired outcome

Blood pressure below 130/85 mmHg

III. Excess weight

1. *Why treat?*

Additional risk factor for the previous conditions

2. *Medications and how to take them*

No medication treatment

3. *What to measure*

Increase aerobic exercise to 30 minutes a day, 3 times a week.

Desired outcome

Weight reduction of 2 lb (1 kg) over the next month

A *Why/How/What* Plan for **Michael's** Medications

I. Diabetes

1. *Why treat?*

Increases the chance of heart disease, kidney disease, blindness, nerve damage, and worsening pain.

2. *Medications and how to take them*

Metformin 850-mg pill. Take by mouth 3 times a day after meals (to minimize stomach discomfort).

Glyburide 5-mg pill. Take by mouth twice a day, 15 minutes before meals (important to eat after taking the pill, to prevent hypoglycemia!)

3. *What to measure*

Home blood test for glucose levels. Take twice a day before breakfast and dinner. Register results in a spreadsheet, present to PCP every 3 months.

In addition, blood test for HbA_{1C} in PCP's office every 3 months.

Desired outcome

Target levels of blood glucose (home measurements): 80 to 130mg/dL.

HbA$_{1C}$ below 7%.

II. Chronic Low Back Pain

1. *Why treat?*

Ruins quality of life. Does not allow you to work full-time and to support family.

2. *Medications and how to take them*

Acetaminophen 1000 mg 3 times a day. Take by mouth at 8 a.m., 3 p.m., and 10 p.m.

Gabapentin 600 mg 3 times a day. Take by mouth at same times.

3. *What to measure*

Daily at 9 p.m.—average pain intensity on that day, on a 0 to 10 scale (0 = no pain; 10 = worst pain I can imagine).

What made pain worse?

What made pain better?

Every Friday: How many daily hours on average I was able to work during the week? Register these in a spreadsheet.

Desired outcome

Alleviate pain enough to be able to work 4 hours a day (probably with pain levels of 3 to 4 on a 0 to 10 scale will be realistic).

After reaching this goal, next goal is to reach 6-hour workday.

III. Excess Weight

1. *Why treat?*

Additional risk factor for heart disease and diabetes. Weight loss can improve glucose control. Excessive weight contributes to back pain.

2. *Medications and how to take them*
   No medication treatment
3. *What to measure*
   Diet: With dietitian Dr. Smith—a plan laid out for meal options for breakfast, lunch, and dinner. No carbonated beverages. No in-between-meals snacks
   Physical activity: Due to current limitation in physical activity—a graded plan laid out
   Current month: 10-minute walk 3 days a week, increase by 5 min/day every 2 weeks
   In 4 weeks: 20-minute walk, 3 times a week
   Long-term goal: 45 minutes of aerobic exercise 3 times a week

Desired outcome
Weigh loss of 3 lb (1.5 kg) over the next 4 weeks

Although the new three-step treatment plan appears to be busier and more complex than the bullet-pointed ones for both Linda and Michael, it is actually the same treatment plan. It has the same overall goals and expectations that were implied in the old treatment plan, but now these two people have formulated clear, specific items to work on. When the outcomes are measurable and have a purpose, they can be more realistically incorporated in your daily schedule, and you, together with your physician, can monitor the treatment success, and make adjustments, if necessary.

Please note that the previous outline does not cover all the components of safe and effective drug therapy—some of these still need to be covered in the following chapters.

Take-Home Message

Taking your drugs properly is not an easy task, and it might be challenging to adjust your drug intake to your daily routine. But remember, drugs work only when taken properly. Having appropriate answers for the three questions outlined in this chapter can be immensely helpful in optimizing your treatment regimen. If your healthcare provider has not specified what each drug is taken for, what is the best way of taking it, and what is the measurable outcome to achieve your treatment goals, it is your responsibility, as a patient, to ask for that information. I stress this point because it is a critical for the success of any drug treatment for any condition.

[6]

AVOIDING UNDESIRED
DRUG EFFECTS

The most common reason people stop taking their drugs or do not adhere to their medication regimen is the experience of **side effects**. And let's agree, it makes a lot of sense. If your painkiller causes terrible constipation, your allergy drug makes you drowsy, or your cholesterol medication causes an annoying headache, you are not very likely to take any of these as prescribed. On the other hand, as we discussed in Chapter 5, if you don't adhere to your treatment, your treatment goals are unlikely to be achieved. Not surprisingly, many patients in this situation feel caught between a rock and a hard place. But let's discuss what the undesired drug effects are and what we can do to minimize them and eventually improve the chances of successful treatment. Some undesired, or adverse, drug effects are unpredictable and thus are difficult to prevent. But research studies estimate that at least 50% of undesired drug events are in fact preventable.

WHAT ARE UNDESIRED DRUG EFFECTS?

As described in Chapter 4, every drug exerts some kind of pharmacologic activity such as blocking an enzyme or activating a receptor.

While we can categorize some of the drug effects as "good" or "bad," "desired" or "undesired," these are all biological effects that are caused by the interaction between the drug and the body. Therefore, the definition of undesired effects (or adverse effects) is somewhat arbitrary. Just to illustrate how arbitrary this definition is, let me give you an example. *Imipramine* is an antidepressant drug—one of the most commonly used drugs to treat depression in the 1970s and 1980s that is still quite widely used. Among the undesired effects of *imipramine* in treating depression is *difficulty in urinating* because *imipramine* binds to certain receptors in the bladder and relaxes the bladder, making urinating more difficult. This is a bothersome side effect for many patients and can sometimes be dangerous, especially in older adults, and many people stop taking the drug because of this effect. On the other hand, for individuals who have urinary incontinence and cannot control their bladder muscles well, which results in frequent and sometimes involuntary urination, *imipramine* is very useful in treating their symptoms. The drug was actually approved by the US Food and Drug Administration (FDA) to treat bed-wetting, and yet bed-wetting has nothing to do with the antidepressant activity; it is the drug's "adverse effect" that is being beneficial in a different group of people. Because this effect on urination is a well-known effect of *imipramine*, the drug should not be prescribed for treating depression to people who have difficulty with urination, for example, men with prostate enlargement.

Side effects of this type that are related to a known pharmacological activity of the drug are also often dose-dependent or concentration-dependent. The higher the drug dose, and consequently the drug concentration at the affected tissue or organ, the higher the likelihood of experiencing these side effects. These effects are typically predictable, as in the example with *imipramine*, and often may be either avoided or minimized.

ALLERGIC REACTIONS

Contrary to side effects related to known pharmacological activity, **allergic reactions** are among universally agreed *undesired* effects and are typically unexpected, unless the person has experienced an allergic reaction to the drug before. The difference between allergic reactions and nonallergic side effects is that allergic reactions are a result of an interaction of the drug with the individual's immune system, rather than as a result of a drug's pharmacological action on certain receptors in target organs. As such, allergic reactions are also not necessarily dose-dependent, meaning that even a small dose can trigger them.

Physicians typically divide allergic reactions to drugs into different types of hypersensitivity, depending on the immunologic mechanism involved. Without getting into the mechanistic details, allergic reactions may present in a wide range of forms. Some are not serious, such as mild itch or sneezing, whereas others can result in moderate skin conditions, such as rash or hives, or serious life-threatening skin reactions. Certain drugs may trigger immune responses that affect the blood, causing, for example, low count of white blood cells (a conditioned called *agranulocytosis*, which would massively increase a person's risk for infection) or platelets (a conditioned called *thrombocytopenia*, which may result in major bleeding). These situation are very rare but may be caused by certain antibiotic drugs or certain antiseizure drugs.

One of the most serious types of allergy, however, is an *anaphylactic reaction* to drugs. An anaphylactic reaction (or *anaphylaxis*) may involve rash, difficulty in breathing, swelling of the tongue and lips, and sometimes additional symptoms such as vomiting and abdominal pain. If not treated in a timely manner, anaphylaxis may send the body into shock, which means lowered blood pressure that does not allow adequate delivery of oxygen to vital organs. This is an emergency situation and requires an immediate intervention by emergency services or in the emergency department. The initial out-of-hospital intervention can be *epinephrine* (self-administration by EpiPen), which by constricting blood vessels reduces the swelling in the airways. If you have had a previous anaphylactic reaction, it is strongly advised that you carry an epinephrine self-injector. The treatment in the emergency department or hospital setting may involve further administration of steroid medications to reduce the inflammatory immune response.

RE-EXPOSURE AND DESENSITIZATION

Once an allergic reaction to a drug has occurred, it is likely that it will occur on the next exposure. Therefore, preventing re-exposure is usually the best way to avoid an allergic reaction to a drug. One important point, though, is that a *rash* or *itch* after taking a drug does not necessarily imply an allergic reaction. Some drugs, including penicillin antibiotics and opioid analgesics, may cause itching or mild rash as a side effect, which will not necessarily occur after an additional exposure. But it is often difficult to differentiate between allergic and nonallergic rash. To be on the safe side, many times the healthcare provider will put a note in the person's record that says, "patient allergic to drug X," even though allergy has not been confirmed.

There may be cases, though, that the treatment is essential, although you may have experienced a previous allergic reaction to it. For example, let's imagine that several years ago you received the antibiotic *vancomycin* but developed an allergic reaction to it. Now you have a serious infection, and the bacteria causing the infection are resistant to many antibiotics, and the laboratory tests show that only treatment with *vancomycin* will effectively kill the bacteria. One way to avoid an allergic reaction (in this case to *vancomycin*) is by *desensitization*. Desensitization procedure will include giving you the "offending" drug in initially a very small dose (sometimes as little as 0.0001% of the therapeutic dose) and then in increasing amounts to allow the immune system to *adapt* to the drug and not cause a hypersensitivity reaction. The desensitization may be done rapidly over several hours for critical drugs and over a prolonged time course with less critical drugs.

CROSS-SENSITIVITY

If you have an allergy to one drug, you may also be allergic to other drugs that have a somewhat similar chemical structure, a phenomenon called *cross-sensitivity*. For example, if you have developed a serious allergic reaction to one type of *penicillin* antibiotic, you are likely to develop such a reaction to other antibiotics in the penicillin family (which includes names such as *ampicillin, amoxicillin,* and others). Moreover, you have about a 10% chance of being allergic to another drug group, called *cephalosporins*, which chemically have a structure somewhat similar to penicillin (see Chapter 20 for further details). The names of these drugs may not end with *cillin* (to ring the bell), but *cephalosporins* include drugs such as *cefuroxime* and *ceftriaxone*.

One possibility to prevent allergic reactions is to avoid these "similar" drugs. But most of you are not organic chemists to figure out whether the structure of your new drug is similar to a drug you are allergic to. This information would typically appear in the drug's leaflet in a form of "don't take this drug if you are allergic to ...." You should also ask your physician or the pharmacist if your previous allergy to a certain drug should prevent you from taking you newly prescribed drug. Even better, if you know you are allergic to drug X, learn what are the drugs to avoid. Cross-sensitivity does not mean that you should absolutely avoid these drugs, but if an effective alternative treatment exists, it is always advisable to choose the less risky option.

Let me provide you with another example. Some individuals have an allergy to *sulfonamide* (or sulfa) drugs. This is sometimes confusing, and people think they will be allergic to anything containing sulfur, but this is absolutely incorrect. It is a certain sulfur-containing structure in the molecule that the immune system reacts to. But various drugs have this structure; for example, if someone has developed an allergy to a sulfonamide-containing drug such as *furosemide* (a water pill to reduce swelling), that person may have an allergic reaction to a *sulfonamide*-containing drug from an entirely different class, for example, *celecoxib* for treating pain (see Chapter 18). Therefore, if you are allergic to *furosemide*, you should learn what other drugs you might be allergic to. You would typically find this information in the drug's label (package insert), which you can always look up online on the FDA's website or find out by asking your healthcare provider. In addition, before taking your newly prescribed *celecoxib*, you should ask your physician or pharmacist if it will be safe to take it given your previous allergy to *furosemide*.

COMMON SIDE EFFECTS AND HOW TO DEAL WITH THEM

Now that we have covered the main points on adverse effects related to allergy, let's get back to pharmacodynamic effects. The most commonly occurring drug side effects are related to gastrointestinal symptoms, like abdominal pain, bloating, nausea, constipation, or diarrhea. These symptoms are quite difficult to tolerate, especially if they last long. For example, one of the most effective drugs for the treatment of diabetes is *metformin* (details given in Chapter 14). *Metformin* helps reduce blood sugar levels and also decreases the risk for various complications such as damage to blood vessels in the kidneys, heart, and eyes. However, *metformin* can cause substantial gastrointestinal side effects. In one of every eight to 10 people treated with *metformin*, the side effects are bothersome enough to cause them to stop the treatment. Side effects such as nausea and bloating are immediately annoying, and even if they are mild, people are not happy experiencing them because the long-term benefits of drugs like metformin are not instantly evident.

This is a tricky situation; we have a wonderful drug that effectively prevents many complications of diabetes, but more than 10% of patients who could have benefited from it refuse to take the drug. You are generally more likely to tolerate unpleasant experiences if you see or expect a clear benefit, or an immediate reward, as outlined in Chapter 5. Since it's quite challenging for most of us to truly appreciate the long-term benefits of treatments such as *metformin*, we are subconsciously less motivated to tolerate the unpleasant side effects. Question 1 from Chapter 5, "*Why* should I take my medication?" comes in pretty handy here; when you realize that the *why* is actually very important to you, the reference point for your motivation can immediately change.

But I am not saying that you need to simply "suffer in silence" with your drugs' side effects for the future benefit. There are various approaches for reducing the severity of adverse effects. For the specific case of *metformin*, dividing the total daily dose to three or four smaller doses instead of two large doses is helpful for some patients. Another possibility is to consult your physician or pharmacist about changing to a different brand. Simply switching to another generic *metformin* (which may have a slightly different release profile or excipient composition) often works well to eliminate or diminish the gastrointestinal side effects. My point is that the fact that you experienced a bothersome side effect should not necessarily lead to stopping an important medication treatment. Try to determine with your healthcare provider how important this treatment is, what the alternatives are, and what approaches exist to overcome some of the undesired drug effects.

Another common reason for discontinuing drug treatment is a "set" of side effects called *anticholinergic effects*. Many drugs cause *anticholinergic* side effects by blocking the receptor to the neurotransmitter **acetylcholine**, which affects many tissues and organs in the body. Most prominent *anticholinergic* effects include dry mouth, blurred vision, drowsiness, and difficulty in urinating (as in the case of *imipramine* I mentioned earlier). These effects are usually dose-dependent as opposed to allergic reactions. Interestingly, most cases of drug discontinuation due to these effects happen when the treatment is initiated at a relatively high dose or the dose is increased too rapidly. Again, once you experience these side effects, it is quite natural that you would not want to continue the treatment. But don't give up at this point.

I want to remind you about the variability that exists among individuals. A "standard" dose that works well for one person may be too high for another person. It is important to remember that for many drugs, especially those prone to *anticholinergic* effects, beginning with doses lower than usual and gradually increasing the dose based on individual response (the process called ***dose titration***) may substantially improve the tolerability of the drug. Let's imagine you are prescribed imipramine to treat depression, with the goal of reaching a dose of 100 mg a day. If you start with that dose, which most of the prescribers will not prescribe, you are VERY likely to develop undesired, especially anticholinergic, effects and stop the treatment immediately. But even if you started at 50 mg or 25 mg a day, you could still develop some of these side effects. At this point, discontinuing the drug and not giving it a "second chance" with a lower initial dose might not be a wise choice, if the drug potentially can be very useful. These situations happen all the time because both initial and target doses of drugs are typically determined based on averages. If, *on average*, a 25-mg initial dose of a drug was tolerable in clinical studies, this could be recommended by the manufacturer and used by clinicians.

As an individual, though, this dose might not be right for you. Let me give you an example of a dose-finding procedure, illustrated in Figure 6.1. In a dose-finding clinical trial for safety (usually called *phase I* clinical trial), the drug is administered in increasing doses. The first participant gets one dose of the drug. If no major side effects are observed, the next participant gets a higher dose. This continues until one participant experiences a side effect, and then the next one receives a lower dose (one level below). If that participant did not report side effects, the next one will again receive a higher dose. By this "up and down" method, a dose that is **tolerable** for **most** of the patients is determined. In Figure 6.1, nobody experienced side effects at the 10-mg dose, and everyone experienced side effects at the 40-mg dose. Above the 25-mg dose (dotted line), two thirds (four out of six participants) reported side effects. Below that dose, six out of eight

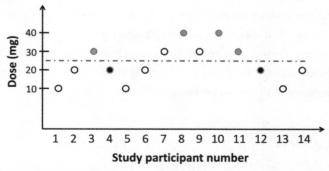

Figure 6.1. Illustration of a dose-finding study in 14 participants. If a participant does not experience a side effect (*white circle*), the next participant receives the drug at the next (higher) dose level. If a side effect is experienced (*gray* or *black circles*), the next participant receives a lower dose. The *dotted line* indicates the dose that was determined as safe in the majority of participants.

participants (75%) did not experience side effect (white circles). This 25-mg dose, then, could be determined by the manufacturer and the regulatory body (e.g., the FDA) as a tolerable dose for *most* patients. However, note that two participants out of eight (i.e., participant 4 and participant 12 [solid black circles]) experienced side effects, which means that even this "tolerable" dose was too high for them.

Again, the variability among individuals pops up as an important factor. In some cases, it is possible to identify these "more sensitive" patients a priori because they may be older adult patients, or those with certain diseases, or those taking certain medications. In many cases, however, the healthcare provider may not be able to predict which individual patient is going to develop a certain drug side effect. My point is that if you started an important drug treatment, but it caused side effects that are known as dose dependent (rather than allergic), instead of stopping the treatment, it might be reasonable to discuss this with your physician and restart the drug at a lower initial dose. For imipramine, for example, some patients need to start at 10 mg a day to tolerate the drug better. As a patient, you are not very likely to know which side effects of the drug are dose-dependent. Therefore, if you have experienced a bothersome side effect of your new medication and are considering stopping the treatment, consult with your physician or the pharmacist. Often there are alternative dose regimens for initiating and titrating your drug in order to overcome many of the initial undesired effects.

WHY NOT ALL PEOPLE SUFFER FROM THE SAME SIDE EFFECTS

The differences in side effects among people consist of many components, similarly to the factors that determine effectiveness that we discussed in previous chapters: age, weight, and genetic differences in drug metabolism (see Chapter 3), for example. In addition, the key elimination organs, such as the liver and the kidneys, play an important role in determining undesired drug effects. If the drug is excreted primarily by the kidneys and they work at 50% capacity, the drug concentration in the blood and various organs is going to be higher than in a person with fully functional kidneys. In these cases, your doctor would probably consider using lower doses or allowing more time between doses (e.g., every 12 hours instead of every 6 hours dosing) to prevent the drug from accumulating in the body. If your kidney function is substantially impaired, you may need to avoid some drugs altogether. Certain blood and urine tests, particularly those assessing the levels of *creatinine*, are useful in determining the extent of kidney function and help to select the appropriate dosing in kidney disease.

People who receive dialysis for their kidney disease have a separate new set of considerations for their drug therapy. Between the dialysis sessions, some drugs are going to stay entirely in the body and are not excreted, potentially increasing their toxicity. In other occasions, the dialysis will eliminate the majority of the drug from the blood in one session and cause a sudden loss of the drug effect. Therefore, it is of critical importance to discuss drug dosing and the need for postdialysis dose supplementation with your nephrologist.

Liver diseases such as hepatitis or cirrhosis may affect liver function and the ability to metabolize drugs. Certain blood tests that assess liver function may help in determining whether drug metabolism is going to be impaired. These tests can guide the decision of using a lower dose or avoiding drugs that are metabolized by the liver.

As I will discuss in Chapters 7 and 8, various foods and drugs may also affect drug pharmacokinetics or pharmacodynamics and increase the likelihood of undesired effects. This also needs to be taken into consideration.

As you can sense, the effectiveness and undesired effects of drugs again boil down to individual differences. Although most drugs that the regulatory agencies approve are considered safe, as Paracelsus wrote in the 16th century, *Dosis facit venenum* (The dose makes the poison)—or in a colloquial form—*every drug is a poison, depending on the dose*. This statement could not be more accurate.

Most people with common sense will understand that taking five pills of the same drug at once for treating headache is probably not a good idea, but in some cases this common sense approach may not be good enough. As we have now discussed on many occasions, it is not always the "dose" that is swallowed or injected that really matters, but rather the "dose" that reaches the various tissues, organs, and receptors in the body. From that standpoint, changes in the pharmacokinetic components of absorption, distribution, metabolism, and excretion (ADME; see Chapter 3) can affect the "dose" that some organs receive.

Some drugs are very safe, and taking five instead of two pills, or taking them while having impaired liver or kidney function, may cause little, if any, damage. Other drugs require a certain range of concentration in the blood to be within the safety margin, and a higher dose (or limited excretion) may have serious consequences. The term **therapeutic index (TI)**, or **therapeutic window**, refers to this safety margin of each drug. The *therapeutic index* is essentially the ratio between the dose that will cause adverse effects and the effective dose. The *therapeutic window* more directly refers to the difference between the toxic and effective blood *concentrations*, rather than doses.

Drugs with a high TI, or wide therapeutic window, are typically safer and can tolerate a larger margin of error without critical consequences. On the contrary, for drugs with a low TI, or a narrow therapeutic window, small changes in doses or blood concentrations may lead to undesired effects. The absolute value of the TI of a drug is less critical; what is important is knowing whether your newly prescribed drug belongs to the **low TI** category, so that you are aware that you need to be extra cautious with any changes or decision regarding the therapy. And this is a question you should refer to your prescribing physician.

It is challenging to cover the majority of low TI drugs in a single book (let alone in a single chapter), but I would like to present three examples of serious undesired effects that can occur with drugs of very different classes. If any of the mentioned drugs are relevant to your condition(s), this section is supposed to give you a sense of what issues to be aware of.

Warfarin (Coumadin, Others)

Warfarin is a drug used for preventing excessive blood clotting, which has a narrow TI (see Chapter 13 for more detailed information). The dose of warfarin should follow a very strict schedule, guided by periodic blood tests for a measure called INR (international normalized ratio—referring to blood clotting) that indicates how much your blood clots. The normal INR values are close to 1, and for most conditions requiring treatment with warfarin, the goal is to increase the INR to a specific range, typically between 2 and 3 (although this may change a bit based on treatment goals, and some people may require a 2.5 to 3.5 INR range to be protected from clotting).

If your INR is below the minimum range, the drug will not protect you from excessive blood clotting, which puts you at an increased risk for a life-threatening blood clot in your heart, lungs, or brain. On the other hand, if your INR is above the upper limit of the range, you are at risk of excessive, potentially fatal, bleeding. Therefore, for effective and safe treatment with *warfarin*, INR measurement and dose adjustments must be performed on a regular basis, and strict adherence to the physician's order is absolutely essential, leaving almost no room for interpretation.

Isotretinoin (Accutane, Roaccutane)

An interesting example of a drug with a delicate balance between desired and toxic effects is *isotretinoin*, a derivative of vitamin A, which is approved for the treatment of *acne*, one of the most common skin conditions worldwide. *Isotretinoin* is taken by mouth daily for 4 to 6 months to treat acne, and it has a tremendously high rate of adverse effects. It causes extreme sensitivity of the skin to sunlight and dryness of skin and various membranes (mouth, nose, eyes), may increase blood cholesterol levels, and may cause liver damage. And if all these are not enough, if *isotretinoin* is taken during pregnancy, it may cause terrible birth defects in the newborn. When one sees this list of potential adverse effects, it is hard to understand why anyone would take such a drug. However, to be fair, *isotretinoin* is an incredible drug because it is one of the rare drugs that can cure a disease, not just provide a temporary or symptomatic relief. Hundreds of thousands of teenagers and young adults who have been suffering from acne have been effectively treated with this drug. The key is that with a good cooperation between the patient and the clinician on appropriate safety measures, the vast majority of patients are safely benefiting from treatment with *isotretinoin*. Changes in liver enzymes and blood cholesterol should be monitored before, during, and after treatment to allow for early detection of problems and therapy modification or cessation, if necessary. Wearing sunscreen (on all exposed skin) on sunny days minimizes the problem with skin hypersensitivity to sunlight. Alternatively, or in addition, the treatment could begin in the autumn, to eventually minimize direct exposure to sunlight. The bothersome effect of dry skin, lips, and eyes is also predictable and is reasonably manageable by applying a moisturizing cream, a lip balm, and eye drops several times a day, as needed. In addition, any woman of childbearing age, if sexually active, is required to use double-barrier contraception methods, such as a combination of condoms and pills, to avoid pregnancy during treatment and up to 3 months thereafter. Despite the relatively narrow therapeutic window, when people responsibly take these precautions, then the treatment becomes less distressing and can be successfully completed with a very reasonable safety margin.

Opioid Analgesics (Morphine, Oxycodone, Hydrocodone, Fentanyl, Methadone)

These drugs are among the strongest painkillers (see Chapter 18 for greater detail), and they all share one particular side effect: they can cause your breathing rate to decrease. This phenomenon is called *bradypnea* [Greek: *bradys*—slow; *pnoia*–breathing], which can be life-threatening because it may cause people to stop breathing. As a consequence, these group of drugs have a relatively low therapeutic index.

When we sleep, our breathing rate goes down because we don't need as much oxygen for activity. But if the amount of oxygen in the blood becomes too low and the amount of carbon dioxide too high, there is a mechanism mediated through our brainstem that urges us to take additional breaths to restore proper oxygenation of the brain and other tissues. Opioid analgesics reduce the sensitivity of nerve cells to painful signals, and they also reduce the sensitivity of certain brainstem nerve cells to carbon dioxide levels in the blood. If the concentration of the opioid in our system is too high, it will cause bradypnea but will also impair the ability to unconsciously compensate for increased carbon dioxide levels by increasing the breathing (respiratory) rate. The result is respiratory depression, and the inability to take in enough oxygen to allow the function of key organs such as the brain and the heart. In fact, respiratory depression is by far the most common cause of death from opioid poisoning or overdose.

In a hospital setting, when patients are closely monitored, reduced breathing rate can be detected by the healthcare personnel, and appropriate drugs to reverse this phenomenon are available (e.g., *naloxone*). However, at home, patients and family members may not notice these changes in respiratory rate until it is too late. Respiratory depression with opioid medications rarely happens when the person is alert and is in substantial pain. It is usually when the person is comfortable and sleepy (or becomes increasingly drowsy) after taking the drug that the respiratory depression occurs. If an opioid-treated person takes less than eight breaths a minute, or becomes unconscious or not responsive, it is an emergency situation that requires *immediate* intervention (i.e., **call 911**). More details are provided in Chapter 18.

Since opioid medication overdoses have reached an epidemic proportion, particularly in the United States, I would like to expand here and demonstrate how the therapeutic window is related to respiratory depression with opioids, which may help prevent some of these cases. We are usually unable to directly measure how much drug there is in someone's brain or brainstem, so blood concentrations of the drug will provide a reference for this example.

Let's simulate how blood concentrations may look in a person who begins treatment with an opioid medication for his or her painful condition. When the person takes the initial first dose (when the blood concentration was zero), the concentration in the blood increases after oral absorption, reaches its highest point (peak), and then declines. The decline rate will depend on several parameters, particularly the drug's *half-life*, which is the time it takes for the blood concentration of a drug to decrease by 50% (see Chapter 4). If the person does not take a subsequent dose, the drug will disappear from the body. It is well-accepted that after five half-lives, there is no substantial amount of drug left in the body. Let's look at the numbers to make sure this concept is comprehensible. Assume we have a drug with half-life of 6 hours, and after we swallow the drug, it reaches a maximum concentration of 160 mg/L in the blood. As you can see in an example in Table 6.1, after five half-lives (30 hours), we will have less than 5% of the initial concentration, which usually is considered negligible.

However, if the next dose of the drug is taken before the previous dose is entirely eliminated, the concentration **builds up** on the remaining amount, and the peak of the second dose will be higher than the 160 mg/L peak of the first dose, and so forth. Typically, this concentration build-up continues for about five half-lives, after which a **steady state** is achieved. The steady state means that with regular dosing, the highest (peak) concentrations and the lowest (trough)

TABLE 6.1 SIMULATED BLOOD CONCENTRATIONS OF AN OPIOID DRUG

Time (hours)	Number of Half-Lives	Concentration (mg/L)	Amount of Drug from Initial Concentration Left in the Blood (%)
0	0	160	100
6	1	80	50
12	2	40	25
18	3	20	12.5
24	4	10	6.25
30	5	5	3.12
36	6	2.5	1.56

concentrations will be in a certain range as long as you take the same doses at same time intervals (as in the last three doses depicted in Figure 6.2). When the drug dose changes, it will again take another five half-lives to reach a new steady state. The ideal situation is that this lowest-to-highest concentration range lies entirely within the *therapeutic window*—that is, above the minimum effective concentration (solid line) but below toxic concentration (dotted line).

The challenge is that no universal *therapeutic window* exists for opioid analgesics because the response and the dose requirements are highly individual. For many other drugs, the concentration range in the window applies to most patients. With chronic opioids, though, each individual will have such a window *of their own at each point in time*. What unfortunately happens is that, sometimes, the analgesic effect is achieved after a few doses, the person continues taking the same dose of drug, but she or he is not aware that the brain and blood concentrations continue to rise because the steady state has not been achieved yet. At a certain point, the drug can reach a

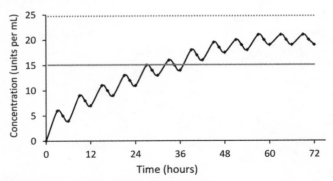

Figure 6.2. Concentration–time curve of a hypothetical drug until reaching the steady state. It took about 48 hours of administration to achieve the steady state with the drug. The therapeutic window lies between the minimum effective concentration (*solid line*) and the minimum toxic concentration (*dotted line*).

critical high enough concentration (above the therapeutic window) to cause respiratory depression and potentially death.

In most cases, serious respiratory depression occurs either within hours or up to several days from initiating therapy or increasing the dose (intentionally or unintentionally). This high-risk time frame also depends on the half-life of the individual opioid medication. The half-life of *methadone*, for example, ranges widely and can be anywhere between 12 and 100 hours. Consequently, if two patients with severe pain came to the same physician, and both were prescribed the same dose of *methadone* as analgesic (e.g., 10 mg 3 times a day), the outcomes might be strikingly different. Methadone blood concentrations can reach a steady state after 2 to 3 days in one of these patients but will keep rising for 2 to 3 weeks before reaching a much higher steady state in the other one, putting that person at a higher risk for serious side effects.

Several approaches to reducing the risk for fatal respiratory depression are available, and I will discuss them in more detail in Chapter 18, but the main principle when initiating treatment with opioids is that during the first few weeks, dose titration should be performed slowly, with the possibility of adding short-acting analgesics if required. You MUST NEVER take opioid doses higher than prescribed. Although one would think that avoiding extra doses is trivial, my experience tells otherwise. When someone is in a lot of pain and has an available prescription medication, the temptation is there to take additional doses to achieve some relief. Unfortunately, with opioids this would be a terrible idea that could have a fatal outcome.

OINTMENTS ARE DRUGS, TOO

One common misconception is that drugs in the form of ointments, creams, or other topical (i.e., local, superficial) applications do not have effects on the whole body, and people therefore tend to ignore prescribing and dosing information. After reading Chapters 3 and 5, it should be quite clear that the skin is a perfectly valid route of delivery of drugs to affect the whole body, similarly to inhalation or administration of rectal suppositories.

If we inject drugs **under** the skin, the drugs will be absorbed in the bloodstream and affect the organism. This is how *insulin* is typically administered in diabetes. When applying ointments or patches **on** the skin, based on the properties of the drugs, they can be absorbed (sometimes substantially) to the bloodstream. Many drugs are indeed intended to act systemically following application on the skin. Certain hormones, such as *testosterone* and *estradiol,* can be delivered through skin patches. Some opioid analgesics, such as *fentanyl,* are delivered through the skin as well. *Nitroglycerine* products for heart conditions and *scopolamine* patches for sea sickness are a few additional examples. However, many people are unaware of this fact when they use topical drugs for a local problem.

For example, topical gels or creams with nonsteroidal anti-inflammatory drugs (NSAIDs) such as *diclofenac* (details in Chapter 18) are commonly used to treat muscle strains, minor traumas, and muscle or joint inflammation. When NSAIDs are taken by mouth or injected, especially at high doses, they may increase the risk for serious side effects such as kidney failure or gastrointestinal bleeding. But even with this knowledge, systemic exposure is often overlooked with topically applied NSAIDs. Unfortunately, several cases have been reported in which people have applied too much of the NSAID gel or cream on a large surface (e.g., the whole back, several times a day, for back pain), which resulted in a huge amount of drug reaching the bloodstream and causing serious problems such as life-threatening stomach bleeding. Some of these were patients with high risk for bleeding, but nevertheless, these unfortunate outcomes could have been prevented if the patients had followed the instructions of maximum recommended dose on the package insert.

Steroid ointments (e.g., *betamethasone, beclomethasone,* and others), applied on large skin areas, can also be substantially absorbed to the bloodstream. When used repeatedly for chronic skin conditions such as psoriasis, systemic side effects of steroids can appear. Although NSAIDs and steroids are probably the exception to the rule rather than the rule, I want to highlight the importance of taking any drug seriously, even if it's "just" a cream or an ointment.

PREVENT HARM TO OTHERS

An additional topic of avoiding undesired drug effects is actually keeping *other* people safe from the undesired effects of *your* drugs. It is your responsibility to keep your drugs in a safe location, for example, far from the reach of children. If you take drugs with a narrow therapeutic index, or controlled substances that have abuse potential, it is of extreme importance that you don't keep them in an accessible area where guests, family members, or occasional visitors to your home can access them. It is especially important if there are teenagers or young adults in the house because they, or their friends, may be tempted to experiment with drugs they can get access to, which has numerous times resulted in serious injuries or death.

SUMMARY

Patients are not expected to understand the pharmacokinetic and pharmacodynamic characteristics of their drugs. It is the prescribing clinician who needs to take these issues into consideration for choosing a safe and effective treatment regimen. However, in the current situation of extremely busy clinics, limited one-on-one time with healthcare professionals, and common use of multiple prescriptions from different providers, some of the safety issues we discussed may go unnoticed. In fact, the undesired drug effects eventually end up resulting in about 1 million hospital admissions and 4.5 million physician office visits every year in the United States alone. As you have seen in the few previous examples, some of these effects can be prevented and managed and need not result in harm, lack of adherence, or treatment discontinuation. In fact, we know from research studies that about 50% of undesired drug effects are **PREVENTABLE**. Your responsibility as a patient is to be alert, to understand that a "one dose fits all" approach rarely works, and to ask the appropriate questions about potential pitfalls of your drugs. Educating yourself about general principles of drug action and the key safety details of the drugs that you take, together with timely discussion of any side effects with your prescriber, are the first step toward more responsible and safe drug therapy.

Take-Home Message

Any given drug may have undesired effects. Some of these effects are unexpected, such as allergic reactions, although some allergic responses can be prevented based on prior responses to drugs and some knowledge of cross-sensitivity between medications. Other effects might be more expected, dose-dependent, and related to the drug's action on its intended or unintended receptor targets. Learning about the factors that affect your drugs' concentration in the blood can help prevent some of the undesired effects of treatment. Understanding dosing principles (starting dose, titration) and proper education on what parameters to monitor can further improve the safety and contribute to the success of your treatment.

[7]

COMBINING DRUGS
WITH FOOD AND DRINKS

Among the most common questions patients ask the pharmacist when filling their prescriptions is whether the medicine needs to be taken on a full or empty stomach. Another popular question is whether there are certain foods or drinks to avoid while taking the drug. Does it really matter? And if it does, what is the reason that some drugs need to be taken on an empty stomach or separated from certain beverages, while others do not? The truth is that for some drugs, it really does not make any difference. For other drugs, this can be a critical determinant of whether the drug will work or not, or whether it will cause side effects. This chapter will provide the reasons and the details of why drugs should or should not be taken with certain foods or drinks.

A patient, whom I met in a community pharmacy, consulted with me regarding her prescription of intravenous (IV) *iron* infusion for treating iron-deficiency anemia. Typically, the infusion is a less convenient, more expensive, and riskier treatment compared with oral *iron* tablets and is reserved for cases in which anemia does not improve with oral treatment. When asked about previous attempts of oral treatment, she responded that her primary care physician prescribed oral *iron* for 2 months, but her hemoglobin level (the blood test that can indicate the severity of anemia) did not improve, hence the decision for IV treatment. We discussed whether she adhered to the oral treatment, and she admitted she simply could not tolerate the *iron* tablets because they caused terrible abdominal pain and constipation. She barely took them for 5 days but never reported this to her physician. She has read that *iron* works better if taken on an empty stomach (which is true), and she took it first thing in the morning. She also usually skipped breakfast, with her first meal being a sandwich around noon.

Indeed, as the package insert suggests, most *iron* products are absorbed better when taken on empty stomach—meaning either at least 1 hour before a meal or 2 hours after a meal, when the stomach is relatively empty. The absorption of *iron* is reduced with food, especially food with high content of calcium, such as dairy products, but also with coffee, tea, and eggs—each inhibiting the absorption of *iron* by a slightly different mechanism. Therefore, ideally, it should be taken on the empty stomach. However, taking *iron* on empty stomach significantly increases the rate of gastrointestinal side effects such as abdominal pain, nausea, and constipation. So here is the dilemma: is it worth trying to take *iron* with food (on full stomach), which is likely to cause less side effects, but understanding that you might not achieve the best possible effect?

After we discussed this issue with her physician, it was decided that she would try another 2 months of oral *iron* therapy, when she takes her *iron* tablets after her sandwich at lunchtime, while refraining from dairy products, tea, and coffee around that time, to minimize the effect on absorption. Indeed, after 2 months she was tolerating the *iron* quite well and was feeling less tired. Her hemoglobin levels improved slower than expected, but within 6 months were much better, and with a very simple treatment modification the patient avoided the need for *iron* infusion treatments.

TAKING DRUGS ON AN EMPTY STOMACH

The absorption of some drugs is negatively, or sometimes critically, affected by food. We just discussed the conundrum of oral *iron* supplements, where improved absorption on an empty stomach may be hampered by gastrointestinal side effects and where an individual decision should be made to achieve a balance between effectiveness and safety.

As with *iron*, some drugs are mostly affected when taken with certain types of food, for example, dairy products. The problem typically is the *calcium* that dairy products contain because *calcium* is a positively charged ion, and when it comes in physical contact with some drugs, it will cause aggregation of the drug molecules (like a magnet pulling tiny metal components to lump together), and they will "sink" in the gut and not get absorbed. For example, some *tetracycline* antibiotics that treat various infections (see Chapter 20) undergo this type of aggregation when taken with dairy products, a process that can reduce their bioavailability by up to 50 to 70%. Nondairy food can still reduce the bioavailability of these antibiotics, but to a lesser extent. The absorption of *doxycycline*, for example, a member of the *tetracycline* group of antibiotics, is less affected by dairy products or food in general (up to 20% decrease), and it can be considered as an alternative. In case you do not tolerate your *tetracycline* on an empty stomach because of side effects, then *doxycycline* could be a better option, if it is appropriate from the standpoint of its antibiotic activity for your infection.

A critical drug-food interaction occurs with the drugs of the *bisphosphonate* family, which are used for treating osteoporosis, preventing fractures, and reducing high blood calcium levels, for example, in certain types of cancer. *Bisphosphonates* keep the calcium in the bones, reducing the "leak" of the calcium from the bones to the blood. Orally taken *bisphosphonates* have very limited bioavailability, some between 0.5 and 2%, which means you may take an oral dose that is 100 times higher than what will eventually reach the blood. About 99% of the dose stays in the intestine, and about 1% (a very precious 1%) gets absorbed to blood to reach the bones and exert its action. These drugs should be taken at least 1 hour before meals (and at least 2 hours after the last meal); therefore, the recommendation is to take them first thing in the morning, 1 hour before breakfast. If taken with or soon after a meal, only about 0.2% of the drug will be absorbed, substantially hampering its activity.

TAKING DRUGS ON FULL STOMACH (AFTER A MEAL)

There are two main reasons some drugs are recommended to be taken on a full stomach. One reason is that some medications have an irritant effect on the stomach and the intestines, somewhat similar to what was described previously for iron. This local irritation may result in abdominal pain, nausea, or diarrhea. Taking the medication on a full stomach can reduce the direct contact between a large amount of drug and the stomach/gut wall and will decrease the irritant effect. Examples of such drugs are nonsteroidal anti-inflammatory drugs (NSAIDs) such as *ibuprofen* and *naproxen* (see Chapter 18) and some antibiotics, which will be discussed in Chapter 20.

The second reason to take certain drugs on a full stomach is that food improves their absorption from the intestine to the bloodstream. Some of the cases pertain to drugs that are lipid-soluble (lipophilic; see Chapter 4). For example, *isotretinoin* for treating acne (Accutane; see Chapter 6) is a lipid-soluble molecule and absorbs better when taken with a meal. In fact, the bioavailability can improve up to two-fold compared with taking the drug on an empty stomach.

The presence of food in the stomach also slows down the absorption of *isotretinoin*, meaning that it is absorbed better but more slowly, preventing side effects associated with high peak concentrations in the blood. Therefore, *isotretinoin* should be taken with meals to help improve the effect as well as the safety margin.

Another, less common case of improved absorption with food relates to drugs that are absorbed into the bloodstream only from the duodenum, a short segment of small intestine immediately after the stomach. When these drugs pass further down the small intestine, they miss the "window of opportunity" to be absorbed. When the stomach is empty, it takes shorter time for a drug to leave it. Therefore, when one of these drugs with a "narrow absorption window" is taken on an empty stomach, it is exposed to the duodenum within a relatively short period, but when the drug has moved past the duodenum, very little further absorption occurs. One of the problems with this kind of absorption is that you get a somewhat abrupt action of the drug, with zigzag highs and lows in blood concentrations during the day. An example of such a drug is *levodopa* for treating Parkinson's disease. Taking it on an empty stomach results in higher peak concentration but in overall lower bioavailability and more erratic response. Taking it with food reduces (flattens) the peak concentration in blood but improves overall absorption and makes the response smoother, with less sharp ups and downs. Another example of a drug with a narrow absorption window is *gabapentin* (Neurontin, others) for treating seizures and certain types of pain. *Gabapentin* is also absorbed mainly from the duodenum, and when the entire dose is quickly released from an empty stomach, only a portion of the taken dose is absorbed. The rest of the dose will "move on," stay in the intestines, and be excreted. Taking *levodopa* or *gabapentin* with food allows these drugs to stay in the stomach longer and "leak" more slowly from the stomach to the duodenum, thus improving the overall bioavailability. A variety of formulations are being developed that will slow down the release of these drugs from the stomach even more, allowing a steadier response and less frequent dosing.

DRUGS TO BE TAKEN WITH A FULL GLASS OF WATER

There are certain drugs that may cause severe irritation to the esophagus (the food pipe) if they come in direct contact with it for long enough time. This may result in ulcers and bleeding of the esophagus. Some people are at a higher risk for such effects, such as patients with anatomical changes in the esophagus and patients with neurological disorders such as stroke. One group of drugs that is problematic from this standpoint is *bisphosphonates* that were just mentioned earlier, although some may be less of an irritant to the esophagus than others. Other groups of drugs that may cause irritation to esophagus include *aspirin* (see Chapter 13), *NSAIDs* for the treatment of pain or inflammation (see Chapter 18), several antibiotics such as *doxycycline* and *clindamycin* for treating bacterial infections (see Chapter 20), *quinidine* for treating malaria and certain heart rate abnormalities, and other medications such as *mycophenolate,* which is used after organ transplantation.

The instructions for taking drugs that can irritate the esophagus are (1) to stand or sit while taking the medication; (2) to take the medication with a full glass of water, beginning with two or three swallows of water before taking the medication; and (3) not to lie down for at least 30 minutes after taking the medication. The idea is to prevent prolonged contact of the drug with the esophagus to minimize irritation. By adhering to these instructions, the overall risk for esophageal damage is very low.

You can imagine that it might be quite cumbersome to take the *bisphosphonates* in the morning, 1 hour before breakfast, with a full glass of water, and not to lie down for at least 30 minutes. However, it is critically important to adhere to these instructions to achieve optimal treatment results, without requiring IV infusions of *bisphosphonates*, which are the alternative for these cases. Because some patients have found it quite difficult to follow this daily ritual, several once-a-week and even once-a-month oral *bisphosphonate* products have been developed; they offer similar efficacy, and you need to go through the "morning ritual" only once a week or once a month. Many people opt for this treatment, but it is more a matter of personal preference. The adherence is not necessarily better with weekly or monthly treatments, it may be more difficult to remember "the *bisphosphonate* day," and missing a weekly or a monthly dose may have more negative consequences than missing a daily dose.

AVOIDING ALCOHOL WHILE TAKING DRUGS

Alcohol may affect drugs in several ways. It may worsen side effects of some drugs; it may affect the blood concentrations of others; and it may cause severe allergic reaction when combined with certain drugs. Because alcohol (or ethanol) can be considered a drug itself, I will describe the combination of alcohol and drugs in more detail in Chapter 8, which deals with interactions between drugs.

AVOIDING GRAPEFRUIT JUICE WHILE TAKING DRUGS

Grapefruit juice has made quite a lot of headlines in the past few years. Taking certain drugs with grapefruit juice may have negative consequences. I would like to provide some details on the topic, which is quite specific to grapefruit—not oranges, grapes, or other fruit.

To understand how grapefruit interferes with medications, we'll need to rely on some of the knowledge from Chapter 3. The enterocytes, which are the cells lining the inner part of the intestine, have various metabolic enzymes such as the cytochrome P-450 (CYP) enzymes that limit the bioavailability of some drugs by breaking them down. Grapefruit (or grapefruit juice) contains compounds that can block these CYP enzymes. Some of these compounds have been identified, called *furanocoumarins*, and include *bergamottin* and similar molecules, while there may still be other unidentified components that are responsible for this grapefruit juice effect.

As you can imagine, if these CYPs in the enterocyte are blocked, less drug will be broken down, and the bioavailability (and blood concentrations) of the drug will increase. As you may recall, the CYP enzymes are located both in the liver and in the gut wall, but in this case, the enzymes in the gut are those primarily affected by grapefruit juice. It is important to note that if a drug initially has close to 100% bioavailability (i.e., is fully absorbed), it cannot be affected much by grapefruit juice because you cannot increase bioavailability beyond 100%. The effect will be relevant mainly for drugs that undergo significant metabolism by the gut CYP enzymes.

Let's take a drug of which, under normal conditions, only 50% would pass the "enzymatic barrier" in the gut wall, and the other half would be broken down. Grapefruit juice will block these gut CYPs, usually for several hours after you had a glass of juice. If you take the drug after drinking the grapefruit juice, this "gut barrier" will not work, and potentially all 100% of the dose will pass to the bloodstream on its way to the liver. And even if some of the drug is metabolized by liver enzymes, the overall *systemic* exposure will still increase. This may cause drug toxicity, which for drugs with a *narrow therapeutic window* can be life-threatening. Table 7.1

TABLE 7.1 DRUGS THAT SHOULD NOT BE COMBINED WITH GRAPEFRUIT
OR GRAPEFRUIT JUICE

Drug Name	Typical Indication (and Potential Risk Due to Interaction with Grapefruit Juice)
Simvastatin (Zocor, others) Atorvastatin (Lipitor, others)	Statin medications—for reducing blood cholesterol levels (interaction may result in muscle breakdown as well as liver and kidney damage)
Sildenafil (Viagra) Vardenafil (Levitra)	Phosphodiesterase 5 inhibitors—for the treatment of erectile dysfunction (interaction may result in low blood pressure)
Verapamil (Calan, Isoptin)	Calcium-channel blocker medication—used to control heart rhythm abnormalities and high blood pressure (interaction may result in very low heart rate and blood pressure)
Felodipine (Plendil, others)	Calcium-channel blocker medication—used mainly for the treatment of high blood pressure (interaction may result in very low blood pressure)
Cyclosporine (Neoral, Sandimmune)	An immunosuppressant drug—used mainly for preventing graft rejection after organ transplantation (e.g., after kidney transplantation) but also used off-label in many autoimmune conditions (interaction may result in kidney damage and toxicity to the nerves)
Clopidogrel (Plavix, others)	Prevents blood clotting—mainly used after heart attack or stroke to prevent recurrence (interaction may result in serious bleeding)

includes a list of medications that are likely to be affected by grapefruit juice intake. The list is not exhaustive but includes drugs for which this interaction can have important consequences. If you are treated with one of these drugs, you should avoid consuming grapefruit juice. Some researchers recommend that consuming the same amount of grapefruit juice every day should be safe with your drugs because no drastic changes are expected in drug blood levels in that case.

It may be wiser, however, simply to eliminate grapefruit (juice) from your diet if you are taking medications that can be affected by it. If you decided that you drink the same amount of grapefruit juice every day with your medications, you may be risking your health with unnecessary side effects of your drugs, should there be a sudden lack of availability of grapefruit juice, for whatever reason.

Grapefruit juice, in addition to blocking CYP enzymes that metabolize drugs, might block some transporter proteins that actually take drugs from the intestine to the blood. In that case, consuming grapefruit juice may actually decrease the bioavailability of the drug by blocking the transporter. One drug, *fexofenadine* (Allegra, for treating allergies), is known to be affected by this mechanism, but other drugs may be identified in the future as well.

Cranberry juice may interact with some blood-thinning medications and increase the rate of bleeding, but it will be discussed in Chapters 9 and 13.

Take-Home Message

Some drugs may not be affected by taking them before or after certain foods or drinks. Other drugs may be quite sensitive to these effects. For example, food may improve the absorption of some drugs but reduce or almost neutralize the absorption of others, particularly if the food has high calcium content. Certain drugs should be taken with food or a full glass of water to prevent local irritation in the gastrointestinal tract. Grapefruit (or grapefruit juice) has components that can inhibit gut wall metabolism of some drugs and increase their bioavailability and potentially their toxicity. You should consult with your physician or your pharmacist regarding the optimal way to take each of your drugs in relation to your meals and certain types of food or drinks. It is usually a good idea to refrain from eating grapefruit or drinking grapefruit juice if you are taking medications on a chronic basis.

[8]

DRUG–DRUG INTERACTIONS

A particularly challenging component in managing drug therapy is the interactions between drugs (also called **drug–drug interactions**). Drug combinations can be anything between harmless and fatal. The issue of drug interactions is of particular concern if your medical conditions are unstable, requiring frequent changes in medications and their doses. Drug–drug interaction occurs when one drug affects the activity of the other. The drugs do not necessarily need to be administered at the same time, or even by the same route. But for a drug–drug interaction to occur, one drug should affect the desired or the undesired effects of the other drug. Sometimes this interaction may result in a positive effect. For example, if you take a caffeine pill with an acetaminophen pill for headache, caffeine will improve the analgesic effect of acetaminophen, even though caffeine alone may not be helpful. However, more often when drug–drug interactions are mentioned, they relate to those resulting in negative, undesired effects. There are several ways by which drugs may interact. Largely, one drug can affect the other drug's pharmacokinetics or pharmacodynamics, as I will describe in detail in this chapter. There is also a small fraction of chemical interactions, in which, for example, two drugs cannot be mixed in an infusion bag because they are chemically incompatible, but I will not discuss those in this book. One does not need to memorize all the different interactions, of course, but understanding the main principles will help you navigate better in the minefield of potentially dangerous drug combinations.

PHARMACOKINETIC INTERACTIONS

Pharmacokinetic interactions can affect any of the four components of the ADME (absorption, distribution, metabolism, and excretion) processes that we discussed in Chapter 3. Let's look at them one by one.

Interactions Affecting Drug Absorption

As we discussed in Chapter 3, a drug that is taken by mouth needs first to be absorbed from the gastrointestinal tract, pass the liver, and then get distributed systemically through the bloodstream. A drug that affects another drug's absorption will cause either an increase or a decrease in the affected drug's bioavailability. An interaction that, for example, affects the absorption of 20% of the oral dose may have very different consequences for different drugs. For drugs that undergo a nearly complete absorption, a 20% difference (let's say a decrease of bioavailability from 90 to 70%, or an increase from 80 to 100%) is not expected to affect you much. On the other hand, for drugs that have low (e.g., 10%) bioavailability, a drug interaction of the same "size" could range from completely blocking the absorption to a three-fold increase (from 10 to 30% absorption) in blood concentration of the drug.

If a drug interaction leads to complete inhibition of a drug's absorption, then "affected" drug will not have any systemic activity. Interactions leading to increased absorption, on the other hand, will increase the chance of experiencing undesired effects. Remember that side effects occur when the drugs reach various tissues, like the brain. As illustrated in Figure 8.1, the brain has no idea what was the initial dose in the pill you took. It can only relate to the fraction of the drug it got exposed to. Therefore, if your heart medication increases the bioavailability of your analgesic drug from 10 to 30%, the brain will not "sense" it as an increase of a mere 20% from the analgesic dose you swallowed. Assuming the blood distribution is proportional to brain distribution, what the brain now sees is a three-fold (300%) increase in drug exposure (see Figure 8.1).

But how can one drug enhance or block the absorption of another drug? Let's look at some of the most common examples. The enhanced absorption is typically similar to how grapefruit juice affects drugs, as we discussed in Chapter 7. You may be taking a drug, a portion of which is normally broken down by cytochrome P-450 (CYP) enzymes in the intestinal wall. If you now take a new drug that

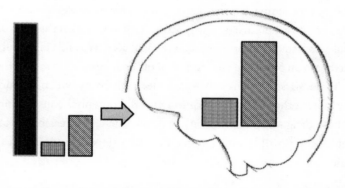

Figure 8.1. Drug A has 10% bioavailability, and the oral dose is 200 mg. That means that from a 200-mg dose (*black bar*), only 20 mg is absorbed (*bar with vertical lines*). If a drug–drug interaction results in increased bioavailability to 30% (*bar with diagonal lines*), the two rectangles may not look substantially different compared with the oral dose (*black bar*). However, for an organ such as the brain (depicted on the *right*), the increase in exposure will be approximately three-fold.

inhibits these CYP enzymes, more of your "old" drug will pass from the intestine to blood because less of it is broken down. The result is more drug in the bloodstream (i.e., increased bioavailability), which means you are going to experience more desired effects but also more side effects. This type of interaction can also occur in the *opposite* direction. Your new drug could *induce* (or enhance the activity of) CYP enzymes in the gut, therefore accelerating the breakdown of your "old" drug as it passes from the intestine to the blood. This will result in a smaller amount of your drug reaching the bloodstream (i.e., decreased bioavailability), which means that you will experience less (desired and undesired) effects from the drug.

Some drugs such as *colestipol* or antacids may chemically bind to drugs that they "meet" in the stomach and cause them to stick together. Since drugs needs to be in their molecular form (floating as single molecules) to get absorbed, this "stuck-together" complex prevents them from being absorbed. Some drugs, by changing the acidity of the stomach environment, may increase or decrease the absorption of certain drugs. Lastly, drugs that slow down the intestine (cause constipation) or increase intestinal activity (and can result in diarrhea) can affect the absorption of other drugs.

Table 8.1 summarizes the main mechanisms by which one drug may affect other drugs' absorption and the potential consequences of these drug–drug interactions. It is, of course, not feasible to present all the possible interactions, but the key is to understand the principle.

Interactions Affecting Drug Distribution

When one drug affects the *distribution* of another drug, it means that the concentration of the "affected" drug in some tissues will change as a result of this interaction. There are several ways one drug can affect another's distribution, but most of these have complex mechanisms,

TABLE 8.1 EXAMPLES OF DRUG–DRUG INTERACTIONS AFFECTING ABSORPTION

Mechanism of Drug Interaction	Selected Examples of "Offending" Drugs	Selected Examples of "Affected" Drugs	Implication of the Interaction
Inhibition of gut wall (enterocyte) CYP enzymes	**Examples of inhibitors**	**Examples of drugs that would be affected**	**Implication of the interaction**
	Ketoconazole (Nizoral), Erythromycin (EES 200), Fluvoxamine (Luvox), Amiodarone (Cordarone)	Cyclosporine (Neoral), Tacrolimus (Prograf), Theophylline (Theo-Dur), Simvastatin (Zocor)	The absorption of the affected drug will increase; the result is higher risk for side effects.
Induction of gut wall (enterocyte) CYP enzymes	**Examples of inducers**	**Examples of drugs that would be affected**	**Implication of the interaction**
	Carbamazepine (Tegretol), Phenytoin (Epanutin)	Cyclosporine (Neoral), Theophylline (Theo-Dur), Warfarin (Coumadin), Simvastatin (Zocor)	The absorption of the affected drug will decrease; the result is reduced effectiveness.

(continued)

TABLE 8.1 CONTINUED

Mechanism of Drug Interaction	Selected Examples of "Offending" Drugs	Selected Examples of "Affected" Drugs	Implication of the Interaction
Change in stomach acidity	**Examples of drugs that can change stomach acidity**	**Examples of drugs that would be affected**	**Implication of the interaction**
	Antacids (Tums, Maalox, Mylanta) Acid-reducing drugs such as omeprazole (Prilosec), lansoprazole (Prevacid), pantoprazole (Protonix) or such as famotidine (Pepcid), cimetidine (Tagamet)	Itraconazole (Sporanox) and ketoconazole (Nizoral) for treating fungal infections, Glipizide (Glucotrol) for diabetes	The effect can be in either direction. For example: *Itraconazole* and *Ketoconazole*: decreased stomach acidity will reduce the bioavailability; risk for loss of effectiveness. *Glipizide*: decreased stomach acidity increases bioavailability; increased risk for side effects such as drop in blood glucose level.

Chemical binding in the gastrointestinal tract	Examples of drugs that can bind other drugs	Examples of drugs that would be affected	Implication of the interaction
	Cholestyramine (Questran), Colestipol (Colestid), calcium, iron, magnesium, aluminum (Maalox, Mylanta)	Furosemide (Lasix) with cholestyramine, ciprofloxacin (Cipro) with aluminum, tetracycline (Acnecycline) with calcium, magnesium, or aluminum	The affected drugs will be less absorbed, and their effectiveness will decrease.

and in this chapter I will provide only one scenario of such type of distribution-based drug interaction, where one drug can change (increase or decrease) the amount of another drug that moves from the bloodstream to the brain.

I mentioned in Chapter 3 that in order to move from the bloodstream to the brain drugs need to cross the blood–brain barrier, which contains *efflux pumps* that can throw out drugs from the brain back to the bloodstream, to protect the brain. A distribution-based drug interaction can occur with medications that inhibit these efflux pumps at the blood–brain barrier. Such an interaction can increase the brain distribution of drugs that would otherwise have limited brain penetration and will thus enhance their undesired effects on the brain. Among commonly used *inhibitors* of these efflux pumps that can increase the brain distribution of other drugs are *clarithromycin* and *erythromycin* (antibiotics), *ritonavir* (for HIV treatment), and *verapamil* (for high blood pressure and heart rhythm abnormalities). The number of drugs that could be affected by this interaction is quite large to list, but if you are prescribed any of the above four drugs, you should ask your physician or pharmacist whether they can interact with other drugs you are taking.

Interactions Affecting Drug Metabolism by *Inhibition*

Probably the most common mechanism for significant drug–drug interactions is when one drug inhibits the metabolism of another drug. As you may remember, CYP enzymes in the liver are responsible for breaking down most drugs, and there are more than 50 different types of CYPs, which are assigned number–letter codes such as CYP3A4 or CYP2C9. Many drugs, by binding to one or more of these CYPs in the liver, can inhibit the activity of these enzymes. The consequence of having such an inhibitor on board is that there are now less CYPs available to break down a drug that would be normally metabolized by that enzyme. This kind of CYP inhibition can cause an increase in the blood levels of the other drug; therefore, the consequences of these interactions can be serious, especially if the "affected" drug has a narrow therapeutic window.

Let's look at an example. John had a stroke as a result of a blood clot in a small blood vessel in the brain. Fortunately, John survived the stroke, but the fact he had such a stroke means that his blood clots excessively and he needs a treatment with an anticoagulant drug that prevents blood clotting, like *warfarin*. Warfarin (discussed in detail in Chapter 13) is effective in preventing the second stroke. On the other hand, *warfarin* is one of the drugs with a narrow therapeutic window, which we discussed in Chapter 7. Warfarin prevents blood clotting but also increases the risk for bleeding. For this reason, John will need to undergo frequent blood tests to ensure the dose he takes maintains his clotting parameters in the desired range. The relevant part to this section is that *warfarin* undergoes significant metabolism by one of the CYP enzymes (primarily CYP2C9). If John is now prescribed a new drug that inhibits the CYP2C9 enzyme (e.g., *fluconazole* for treating a fungal skin infection), the metabolism of *warfarin* is going to be impaired, leading to higher blood concentration and increased risk for major bleeding. Thus, we have an example of a drug–drug interaction that needs to be avoided.

In general, the key is in *identifying the potential interaction BEFORE it happens*, before the "offending" drug is prescribed. If the "offending" drug is necessary, frequent monitoring and dose adjustments by the prescribing physician can minimize undesired effects. But for high-risk drugs such as *warfarin*, if such a CYP-inhibiting drug is prescribed and dispensed unnoticed, the patient's life would be at risk. In fact, I recently evaluated a patient who was co-prescribed warfarin and *fluconazole* by two different physicians, and it was a matter of luck that we identified the interaction before major bleeding occurred. The blood tests showed that the interaction had resulted in her bleeding parameters exceeding twice the recommended maximum.

Therefore, for each of your medications, it is important that you verify the compatibility of the drugs with your physician or pharmacist every time a new prescription or over-the-counter drug is started or stopped. And at the very least, you should share what other medications you are taking when a new drug is prescribed. The issue is also important when you stop a medication that you have been taking for a while. If the CYP enzyme has been chronically inhibited by a drug you have been taking and you have now stopped taking it, the enzyme activity will increase, and it can affect other drugs' metabolism.

Interactions Affecting Drug Metabolism by *Induction*

Induction of liver enzymes is a process in which a drug increases the amount of drug-metabolizing CYPs available in the liver. If *drug A* is metabolized by a CYP, and you add *drug B*, which is an *inducer* of that CYP, then *drug A* is going to be broken down more rapidly. The outcome is the exact opposite of CYP inhibition that I described in the previous section with warfarin; this results in *drug A* being eliminated at a higher rate, and its blood concentrations will decline. In many cases of induction-based interactions, no imminent danger occurs to the patient. The usual result is that *drug A* is now not efficacious enough, but then by increasing the dose, it might be possible to compensate for the extra amount of drug that is metabolized because of enzyme induction. This approach of dose adjustment is mainly relevant in conditions in which we have a clear measurable outcome. For example, if the "affected" *drug A* is an analgesic, you will experience more pain, and the dose of the analgesic can be increased to provide sufficient relief. Similarly, if *drug A* is for treating high blood pressure, we could measure your blood pressure and adjust the dose accordingly.

In some cases, however, this adjustment is quite challenging if it refers to disease prophylaxis or the prevention of certain conditions or events. For example, if your treatment is given to prevent a heart attack, you will not know if this treatment has been truly effective until you have a heart attack. If you have undergone a kidney or lung transplantation, you will need immune-suppressive drugs for preventing your immune system from rejecting the precious transplant (the graft). Unless blood levels of the immunosuppressant drug are carefully monitored, you will not know if an enzyme-inducing drug interaction is causing reduced blood levels of your post-transplantation medication. This situation can impose substantial morbidity risk. The important message here is that if you receive a medication for preventing a condition, whether it is for preventing a heart attack, stroke, pregnancy, infection, or organ rejection, you must be very attentive to any newly prescribed medication and check with you doctor or pharmacist to make sure that the new drug does not reduce the effectiveness of your preventive medications. Importantly, this enzyme induction process takes time, and maximum inducing effect may occur 2 to 3 weeks after the "offending" drug has been initiated.

A few years ago, I had a patient who came to the pain clinic with severe pain after shingles (herpes zoster). She had undergone a lung transplantation a few years before and was treated with, among other drugs, an immunosuppressant drug called *tacrolimus* (Prograf) for preventing her lung transplant rejection. A week before coming to the pain clinic, a primary care physician had prescribed *carbamazepine*, one of the drugs that can help treat the pain from shingles (see Chapter 18). There are several drugs that could have been used for that purpose, but *carbamazepine* was actually quite a poor choice in her case because it is a very strong **inducer** of CYP3A4, which metabolizes *tacrolimus*. The patient had not felt any change related to tacrolimus effect, but we immediately sent her to the lab to obtain blood levels of tacrolimus, and the results showed that the concentration had dropped by 40% from her previous result and was now below the "therapeutic window" for effective prevention of graft rejection. Her *carbamazepine* was discontinued, her *tacrolimus* dose was temporarily increased (because it takes some time for CYP enzymes to get back to their baseline activity), and luckily her recovery was uneventful. She did get a different treatment that helped her with her shingles pain that did not interact with her medications.

This is a classic case in which the prescriber should have been more careful in prescribing her new medication and should have checked for potential interactions. Unfortunately for the patient, her primary care physician was on vacation the week she presented with shingles, and in fact it was a different physician, who was less familiar with her medical history and prescribed the *carbamazepine*. My point is that these cases may happen, and blaming bad luck is not going to help. People who take such important medications should be aware that serious drug interactions may critically affect their therapy and scrutinize every newly added drug. *Carbamazepine* is one of those classic "offenders" that can reduce the efficacy of immunosuppressant drugs by enzyme induction. There are several drugs in this category of liver enzyme inducers, but the most significant interactions occur with drugs used for the treatment of seizures, such as *carbamazepine* (which is also used for nerve injury pain), *phenytoin*, and *phenobarbital*, some antibiotics such as *rifampicin*, and HIV drugs such as *efavirenz* and *nevirapine*.

Interactions Affecting Drug Excretion

Excretion through the kidneys to urine is one of the major processes of eliminating drugs from the body, as mentioned in Chapter 3. What is eliminated can be the drug itself (what is called the *parent drug*) or the products of the drug's metabolism in the liver (i.e., the *metabolites*). These metabolites can be inactive, active, or sometimes toxic. The removal of a drug from the blood through the kidneys mainly involves processes mediated by transporter proteins that move the drug from the blood to urine. Once in the kidney, however, the drug, in a passive diffusion-like process, can be reabsorbed back to the blood. Because of this bidirectional balance, the eventual elimination of drugs to urine can be increased or decreased by drug–drug interactions affecting these two processes of transporter-mediated drug excretion and passive drug reabsorption.

Let's assume that *drug A* is excreted by the kidneys. If *drug B* competes with *drug A* for the same transport mechanisms of excretion, it may inhibit the excretion of *drug A* to urine. If both drugs are taken over time, the blood concentrations of *drug A* will rise.

Probenecid (for treating certain types of arthritis) can reduce the kidney excretion of *methotrexate*—which is a drug used for treating many types of inflammatory and immune conditions. Combining both drugs will result in toxicity of methotrexate. *Quinidine* (for treating malaria and heart rhythm abnormalities) can increase the toxicity of *digoxin* (used for treating heart failure) by the same mechanism. Note that both *digoxin* and *methotrexate* are drugs with a narrow therapeutic window; therefore, changes in blood concentration will have important clinical implications.

The passive excretion rate mainly depends on the physicochemical properties of a drug. It can be affected by the acidity (pH) of the urine. Some drugs can increase the acidity of the urine (e.g., *vitamin C*) or decrease the acidity of the urine (e.g., *bicarbonate*—baking soda), which will affect the reabsorption of certain drugs. Among the important pH-changing interactions are those between diuretic drugs (water pills) and *lithium*, which is a drug used for treating certain mental health conditions such as bipolar disorders. Additionally, prolonged use of various antacids, especially those containing magnesium and aluminum salts, may decrease the urine acidity and accelerate the excretion of aspirin and other acidic drugs into urine, overall reducing their effectiveness.

PHARMACODYNAMIC INTERACTIONS

Now that we covered main types of pharmacokinetic interactions, which affect the drug movement and concentration in the body, let's look at pharmacodynamic interactions. Pharmacodynamic interactions are primarily based on one drug enhancing the effect (or toxicity) of another drug, or reducing its activity, without changing its blood concentrations. These types of interactions are less well-studied than pharmacokinetic interactions because it's more difficult to quantify them owing to lack of measurable changes in drug concentrations. Nonetheless, they exist, and many are of clinical importance. The good news is that pharmacodynamic interactions are easier to anticipate because either the drugs have pharmacologic (desired or undesired) activity "in the same direction" and their combination will enhance this effect, or they have antagonistic activity "in the opposite directions," and one will diminish or neutralize the effect of the other drug. However, this "anticipation" involves being familiar with the desired and undesired effects of each of your drugs.

Interactions "in the Same Direction"

The most trivial example would be combining two drugs to treat the same condition. If each drug reduces blood pressure by a different mechanism, their combination may result in a desirable interaction: that the blood pressure will be reduced more than with each individual drug. On the other hand, the combination may reduce the blood pressure too much and cause dizziness, but that would be an expected effect that could be managed by adjusting the drug doses.

Let's consider expected undesired effects like the combination of *opioid analgesics* and *benzodiazepine hypnotics*. As we described in Chapter 6, opioids may cause drowsiness and respiratory depression. *Benzodiazepines* (i.e., drugs such as *diazepam* [Valium] or *lorazepam* [Ativan]), which are mostly used to treat anxiety and insomnia, also increase the risk for both drowsiness and respiratory depression, although they act at different receptors than opioids. It is therefore not surprising that the combination may increase the risk for these side effects even further. Indeed, there is an increased risk for death due to respiratory depression if you combine an opioid with a benzodiazepine. The risk for respiratory depression is even higher if you have a chronic lung disease; therefore, the individual clinical condition, as well as the drug dose, would be important in deciding the potential severity of the interaction.

A bit more complex example would be the addition of side effects that are not intuitive. If you are taking *quetiapine* (Seroquel) for a mental health condition, it may somewhat increase the risk for a certain type of arrhythmia—heart rhythm abnormalities. Typically, if you don't have a heart condition, you would be at a low risk for such a side effect and would likely not experience changes in heart rhythm. However, if you now have a urinary tract infection and are prescribed an antibiotic, *ciprofloxacin* (see Chapter 20), which also can increase the risk for the same side effect, your overall risk for arrhythmias increases as a result of combining both drugs. Although this interaction is less intuitive than the one with two blood pressure medications or the *opioid-benzodiazepine* combination, it is still predictable, and the prescribing clinicians should be aware of the side effects of drugs they prescribe. But as I stressed many times before, double-checking before filling your prescription would be important for preventing an undesired drug–drug interaction in such a case.

Interactions "in the Opposite Directions"

When you learn about what your drug does, as well as what side effects to expect, it also becomes possible to anticipate drug–drug interactions based on antagonistic effects of drugs. You would probably avoid drinking a strong espresso before you go to bed if you typically take a sleeping medication to fall asleep. The logic behind drug interactions in this category is the same. If one drug causes diarrhea and the other causes constipation, if one drug increases the heart rate and the other decreases the heart rate, they will negatively interact, based on their pharmacodynamics.

Some mechanisms behind these interactions are less obvious than a change in heart rate or alertness because the "effect" may not be as easily recognizable. Then, the information described in Chapter 4 for understanding how your drug works becomes important. *Warfarin,* for example, is a blood thinner that works by inhibiting a certain step of *vitamin K* activity in the body (see Chapter 13). Taking *vitamin K* will contradict, or antagonize, the activity and the clinical effect of *warfarin*. In fact, *vitamin K,* because of this pharmacodynamic interaction, is what you would receive in the hospital to treat an overdose of *warfarin*.

More rarely, pharmacodynamic interactions may result in counterintuitive results. The blood-thinning effect of aspirin is caused by its binding to a certain enzyme in platelets to prevent blood clotting. Aspirin has a short half-life in the blood, but once it binds to a platelet, it permanently and irreversibly neutralizes it, allowing the use of once-daily low doses (what is called *baby aspirin*) to prevent heart attacks. *Ibuprofen* (Advil, Nurofen), a popular analgesic and anti-inflammatory drug, also binds to the same platelet enzyme, so you would expect a similar or enhanced pharmacodynamic effect from the interaction between *aspirin* and *ibuprofen*. However, unlike *aspirin, ibuprofen* detaches from the platelet after a few hours. If *ibuprofen* is taken within 1 to 2 hours **before** taking aspirin, *aspirin* will not be able to exert its full long-term activity because the enzyme is "busy" binding *ibuprofen*. The details are described in Chapter 13, but this is a very common drug combination and is probably worth mentioning an additional time.

SMOKING AND ALCOHOL

Although we are focusing primarily on medications, smoking and alcohol consumption may also affect other drugs you take. Alcohol (ethanol) can be considered a drug itself; smoking delivers nicotine and a variety of chemicals to our body, and these can affect other drugs' pharmacokinetics and also pharmacodynamics.

Smoking

If you smoke but care about your own health and about the health of the people around you, then you should quit. I do not intend to imply it is simple to quit smoking, but there are certainly behavioral and medical approaches that can help. In addition to the known numerous direct health hazards of smoking, you should also be aware of how smoking may potentially affect drugs you might be taking. Chronic smoking induces some of the liver enzymes, especially CYP1A2, and the effect will be similar to taking a liver enzyme–inducing drug as described previously.

Several drugs, including *theophylline* for treating asthma (see Chapter 15), *mexiletine* for treating arrhythmias, *duloxetine* for treating depression (see Chapter 17) or nerve injury–related pain (see Chapter 18), and *olanzapine* and *clozapine* for treating schizophrenia, are all affected by smoking. In all these cases, smoking will induce CYP enzymes and decrease the blood concentration, and thus the effectiveness, of these drugs. Interestingly enough, patients with schizophrenia are among those with the highest smoking rates in the world (60 to 70% are smokers), and some of the major antipsychotic drugs are not going to work well for them (or require higher doses and cause more side effects) because of smoking.

For people who smoke and take chronic medications: if you plan to quit, consult with your doctor or pharmacist about whether any of your drugs could have been affected by your smoking. Removing the "enzyme-inducing" effect of smoking may require dose adjustment of some drugs to prevent increased effect or toxicity of medications that are affected by smoking.

Alcohol

Alcohol may interact with various drugs in four different ways:

1. *Disulfiram-like reaction.* Combining some drugs with alcohol can cause a serious intolerance (or allergic-type) reaction, which includes severe flushing, vomiting, headache, increase in heart rate, and low blood pressure. Some of the drugs that can cause such a reaction when taken in parallel with alcohol include antibiotics such as *metronidazole* (Bactrim), *tinidazole* (Tindamax), and certain *cephalosporins* (see Chapter 20); some antidiabetic medications such as *glyburide* (Micronase) and *glipizide* (Glucotrol); and some cardiac drugs such as *nitroglycerin* (Nitrostat, Nitrolingual). It is impossible to predict whether you would experience such a reaction if you combined your drug with alcohol. Therefore, alcohol is best avoided at least 24 hours before and after taking these medications.

2. *Inhibition of liver enzymes—acute alcohol consumption.* Alcohol is metabolized by liver CYP enzymes. Consumption of

moderate alcohol amounts with other drugs that are metabolized by CYPs can compete for the enzymes and result in increased concentration (and toxicity) of other medications.

3. *Induction of liver enzymes—chronic alcohol consumption.* In people who consume moderate to high amounts of alcohol on a daily or almost daily basis, CYP activity is induced, similarly to chronic smokers. In this case, drugs that are metabolized by various CYPs may become less effective. In the case of acetaminophen, in which toxic metabolites are produced by CYP metabolism, even more toxic metabolites will be produced in chronic drinkers, resulting in higher risk of liver damage. In general, chronic alcohol drinking increases the risk for liver disease, and the combinations with drugs that can cause liver toxicity may further increase this risk.

4. *Additive side effects.* Alcohol, even in moderate amounts, can cause drowsiness and impaired motor skills and coordination. There are multiple drugs that may cause similar effects, mainly those working in the central nervous system—drugs such as benzodiazepines (*diazepam, clonazepam*), antihistamines (*diphenhydramine, chlorpheniramine*), antidepressants (*amitriptyline, clomipramine*), opioid analgesics, and muscle relaxants. Combining these drugs with alcohol is likely to increase the severity of those side effects and can lead to injuries due to accidents and falls.

Combining alcohol with some medications for treating diabetes (e.g., *glipizide* and *glyburide*) may increase the risk for *hypoglycemia*, which is a drop in blood sugar levels to below the normal range.

Many online resources and databases are available to check drug–drug interactions, but for a nonprofessional it may be difficult to assess the reliability of the information. Moreover, for each person, the importance and the clinical relevance may differ. However, being proactive and being educated about potential interactions of your drugs may be a good idea. One of the worrying findings about drug interactions is that in a given year, one of every 35 people older than 50 years is inadvertently prescribed a combination of two or more drugs that is dangerous or contraindicated (i.e., the drugs *must not* be prescribed to the same patient at the same time). This does not refer only to people who take chronic drugs; it's one out of every 35 adults who are prescribed any medication. So as I have highlighted before, the responsible actions would be to find out whether your drugs have a potential for interactions and to be diligent about likely negative outcomes. Now that, after reading this chapter, you are familiar with possible mechanisms of drug interactions and with concepts such as enzyme *inhibitors* and *inducers,* it will be easier for you to interpret information on drug interactions that you read or hear about from your provider. By learning the key drug–drug interaction details relevant to your drugs, you can anticipate and help prevent negative or harmful outcomes of drug interactions.

Take-Home Message

Many drugs negatively interact with each other, resulting in either reduced effectiveness or excessive undesired effects. The interactions by large can be divided into pharmacokinetic and pharmacodynamic. The pharmacokinetic interactions refer to situations in which one drugs affects the absorption, distribution, metabolism, or excretion of another drug. Depending on whether the net effect is an increase or decrease of a drug's blood concentration, the direction of the interaction can be estimated. Although many drugs interact on this basis, these interactions mainly have serious consequences for drugs with low *therapeutic index.* The interactions that result in decreased drug effect are challenging in terms of preventative interventions because they may go unnoticed until the event (that was supposed to be prevented) occurs. It is important to consider interactions not only when adding a new drug but also when discontinuing a drug that you used to take chronically.

Pharmacodynamic interactions "make more sense" because they usually result from combining drugs with similar actions (and then the result is augmentation of the pharmacological effect) or opposite actions (in which case the net result is reduction of the desired effect). It is also important to note that alcohol and smoking may interact with drugs, and using (or stopping) either can affect your medications.

[9]

DO IT YOURSELF

Over-the-Counter Drugs
and Disease Prevention

You are probably not overly enthusiastic to visit your doctor's office, even when you really have to. Indeed, most people prefer taking care of themselves if they can. A substantial portion of this *taking care of yourself* process involves taking nonprescription medications and making day-to-day decisions about your lifestyle for preventing illness. This chapter will touch on these two areas where you are likely to make independent decisions: (1) the use of nonprescription drugs and dietary supplements, and (2) routines for disease prevention.

OVER-THE-COUNTER MEDICATIONS

Although the majority of drugs require prescription, many drugs are available over the counter (OTC). The OTC designation means that these drugs can be obtained without a prescription, either from the pharmacist or directly from the shelf in a self-service area of a pharmacy or in grocery stores or gas stations licensed to sell OTC drugs.

There are more than 300,000 marketed OTC products in the United States, across dozens of therapeutic classes of drugs, such as analgesics, antacids, sleep medications, and acne products. This chapter cannot possibly discuss the potential advantages and risks of all OTC drug classes, but it is important to highlight some of the key issues that you need to know before initiating treatment with OTC drugs. As with prescription medications, safe use of OTC drugs requires some knowledge and, more important, personal responsibility for the drugs you purchase without a prescription.

Generally, OTC drugs are drugs that have been found to be safe and appropriate for use without the supervision of a healthcare professional. Although they are generally safe, it does not necessarily mean that they are safer than prescription medications in the same class—nor does it mean they are safe for everyone. In fact, the use of some OTC drugs requires extreme caution because they may cause harm if not taken properly. I quoted Paracelsus in an earlier chapter—*every drug is a poison, depending on the dose*. This is particularly important in the setting of OTC drugs consumption because the responsibility lies solely on you; there is no additional level of protection or a control barrier in the form of advice from a healthcare professional, *unless you ask for that advice*.

One important point I would like to make is that OTC medications are considered **safe** within the *dosage range indicated on their label*. If the label reads take up to two pills 3 times a day (i.e., overall six pills a day), the patient generally has no further information about what might be a harmful dose—eight, 10, or 16 pills. Therefore, if the recommended dose and length of treatment as indicated on the label do not help with your symptoms, increasing the dose or the treatment duration on your own is often a bad idea. This is the time to consult a healthcare professional.

This brings me to one of the most important components of OTC drugs—**the label**! Unless you have read the label, you probably won't know what are the recommended maximum dose and duration of treatment. So please, READ THE LABEL carefully!

The label will include information about the drug class and its medical **use** and, more important, **warnings** that describe who should not take the medication and what **side effects** the drug can cause. The label will also include the **directions** for properly taking the medication, appropriate **storage** conditions, and any inactive ingredients. If you have **allergies,** make sure you are not allergic to any of the *active* or *inactive* ingredients of the drug before taking it. An active ingredient (compound) refers to the molecule that exerts the intended pharmacological effect, such as *acetaminophen* in Tylenol products. Inactive ingredients refer to compounds added to the drug product to give it a shape, color, taste, and help with easier swallowing and break down in the stomach or intestine. They are typically neutral and do not have effects of their own. However, their list always appears on the package insert, and it's useful for checking for potential allergies.

Although OTC medications are perceived as safe, some are among the most highly abused drugs in the Western world. In fact, The National Institute of Drug Abuse reports that more people in the United States abuse OTC cough medicines, particularly drugs containing *dextromethorphan,* than *cocaine.* The abuse, or *misuse,* to use the more appropriate term, is related to the use of doses that are much higher than indicated, at which some drugs may have pleasurable effects and addictive properties. But higher doses are also much more likely to result in side effects and damage to various organs, such as the liver, the kidneys, or the brain. The use of OTC drugs *as labeled, and by the consumer to whom the drug is intended* will essentially prevent inappropriate use. This again, as mentioned in Chapter 6, highlights the importance of making sure that other people do not have access to your drugs and the importance of not sharing your drugs with other individuals—because the drug that is safe for you might not be safe for someone else.

There are several considerations when choosing a safe OTC drug, so I will divide the discussion into two sections. First, I will deal with a few examples of OTC medications and discuss the scenarios in which they are **not appropriate** or potentially harmful. Second, I will look at OTC drugs from a different perspective, discussing certain medical conditions that can put you at higher risk for undesired effects of OTC drugs. Although there will be some necessary overlap between these sections, it's important to focus on both questions— "Which OTC drugs should I be extra careful about?" and "Which of my existing medical conditions I should be concerned with when choosing an OTC drug?"

COMMON OVER-THE-COUNTER MEDICATIONS

Painkillers (Analgesics)

The most commonly used painkillers are acetaminophen (*paracetamol*) and various nonsteroidal anti-inflammatory drugs (NSAIDs). Some *NSAIDs* are available by prescription only, but lower doses of many of these are available OTC.

Acetaminophen is one of the most commonly used drugs in the world. It is usually safe, but it is very important that you stick to the recommended dose and keep it away from children. For an adult, the total daily dose should not exceed 4000 mg (4 grams). *Acetaminophen* overdose may cause serious, and sometimes fatal, liver damage. Another point to remember is that *acetaminophen* is very common in combination products for treating flu and cold. You need to make sure you do not exceed the 4000-mg dose limit from ANY *acetaminophen*-containing products combined. You should be extra careful with *acetaminophen* if you have liver disease and consult your physician or pharmacist on the appropriate dose.

Several NSAIDs such as *ibuprofen* (Advil, Motrin), *naproxen* (Aleve, Naprosyn), and *aspirin* can be obtained without a prescription. In doses higher than recommended, these drugs will increase your risk for serious stomach or intestinal bleeding. This risk is especially high if you are older than 65 years, if you suffer from stomach or intestinal ulcers, or if you have experienced prior intestinal bleeding. In addition, the bleeding risk increases when NSAIDs are combined with blood thinners, corticosteroids (for treating inflammation), or selective serotonin reuptake inhibitor (SSRI) antidepressants (see Chapter 17). Do not use NSAIDs without consulting your physician if you have kidney disease, diabetes, or asthma. Recently, the US Food and Drug Administration (FDA) issued a warning that prolonged use of NSAIDs is associated with increased risk for heart attack and stroke. In general, NSAIDs are wonderful drugs when used at recommended doses for short periods of time but can have devastating effects if used incorrectly.

Some products include both *acetaminophen* and *aspirin* (e.g., Excedrin); therefore, both sets of the previous precautions apply to these products.

Allergy, Flu, and Cold Medications

Many products exist for treating cold and flu; some of them contain a single active ingredient, but many are combination products. Because some contain *acetaminophen* or an NSAID (mentioned previously), the precautions of these analgesics will apply to these cold and flu products. Other common ingredients are *antihistamines* and *decongestant drugs*.

Antihistamines (e.g., *chlorpheniramine* and *diphenhydramine*) are present in many products like Chlor-Tabs, Benadryl, and Triaminic. Antihistamines may cause drowsiness and impair driving ability and concentration. Avoid taking antihistamines with alcohol, with other sedating drugs (e.g., drugs for treating anxiety), and with opioid analgesics because they can worsen each other's side effects. Don't take OTC antihistamines if you have a seizure disorder because they may increase the risk for seizures. Antihistamine medications may cause anticholinergic effects (see Chapter 6 for a refresher); therefore, combining with certain medications such as antidepressants can worsen these side effects.

Decongestants, also called *sympathomimetics*, such as *pseudoephedrine* and *phenylephrine* (Sudafed, Triaminic Cold and Allergy) are often found in what are labeled "nondrowsy" cold medications. These drugs, especially at higher doses, may increase blood pressure and heart rate. Therefore, they can cause problems in individuals with high blood pressure, in people with heart disease, and in people taking drugs for the heart or high blood pressure. Decongestants come in oral formulations and also in nasal sprays; oral formulations might be more effective but have higher risks for side effects. Both with oral and nasal routes of administration, prolonged use is not recommended because it can cause a "rebound effect": the swelling of mucous membranes (which initially caused congestion) after the drug effect wears off, requiring you to use more of the medicine.

Blood Thinners

Aspirin is an NSAID available OTC. Although doses of 250 mg and higher are used in products for managing pain and fever, low doses (usually between 75 and 100 mg a day) are used to prevent blood clotting, as described further in Chapter 13. Since low-dose *aspirin* has been effective in preventing heart attacks and strokes in patients with risk factors such as diabetes and heart disease, many people decide to take *aspirin* without having a prescription or a recommendation from their physician. Despite the demonstrated effectiveness of *aspirin* and its availability as an OTC drug, it is best to discuss with your doctor *if* aspirin is good for you. You should be very diligent and understand the risks associated with *aspirin*, which are primarily related to increased risk for bleeding, especially if you have other risk factors for bleeding or take drugs that can potentially interact with *aspirin*.

Cough Medications

Several groups of cough medications are available without prescription. Some of them mainly help with dry cough (i.e., depress the cough reflex); others are used mainly for treating productive ("wet") cough because they reduce mucus thickness and help get rid of mucus faster. Similarly to antihistamines, cough medications also come in a variety of combinational cold and flu products. Remember, medications containing *dextromethorphan* (Theraflu, Delsym, and others) can have abusive potential when used on regular basis with doses exceeding the ones that appear on the label. In many countries, some of the nonprescription dry cough medications include *codeine*, which is a weak opioid and at larger doses has abuse potential as well. Another medicine for productive cough, available without prescription in many countries, is *promethazine*. *Promethazine* is quite safe when administered in low doses, but at high doses, especially in children, it may cause heart rhythm abnormalities. It is also important to pay attention to the alcohol content in some cough and cold syrups and to limit the amount of intake, especially in children.

Orlistat

Orlistat is a medicine for reducing weight, which has been approved by the FDA as an OTC product (Alli). *Orlistat* promotes weight loss by reducing the absorption of fat from food. However, it appears that orlistat interacts with a significant amount of drugs, and people considering the use of orlistat should be aware of it. For example, orlistat may substantially decrease the effect of several drugs used for treating epilepsy and may reduce the absorption of thyroid hormones.

Orlistat may increase the risk for bleeding if you take the blood thinner *warfarin*. As I mentioned in Chapter 8, *vitamin K* opposes the effect of warfarin, and since *Vitamin K* is a fat-soluble vitamin, prolonged use of orlistat may decrease it absorption from food (because it decreases the absorption of a variety of fatty molecules), which will eventually enhance the effect of warfarin.

MEDICAL CONDITIONS REQUIRING EXTRA CAUTION WITH OVER-THE-COUNTER DRUGS

If you have certain medical conditions, you should be extra careful when choosing an OTC drug. Table 9.1 provides examples of several common conditions and the issues associated with using OTC drugs if you have these conditions. As a rule of thumb, if you have ANY chronic conditions or take multiple medications, you should ask your doctor or consult your pharmacist *before* taking OTC drugs.

COMPLEMENTARY AND ALTERNATIVE MEDICINE

Natural supplements, vitamins, and herbs (collectively a part of *complementary and alternative medicine*, or CAM) are a group of products that can be used without direct physician's supervision. Some of them meet the criteria of OTC products, and some don't. Regardless, they all are available for purchase without a prescription. These products warrant separate attention because some of them have proven benefits for certain conditions while others have claimed benefits.

TABLE 9.1 COMMON CONDITIONS AND ASSOCIATED INAPPROPRIATE
OVER-THE-COUNTER MEDICATIONS

Conditions	OTC Medications that May Not Be Appropriate
Liver disease	Acetaminophen is dangerous. Certain antihistamines and NSAIDs may be dangerous. Consult with healthcare professional before any OTC product use.
Kidney disease	NSAIDs are dangerous. Consult with healthcare professional before any OTC product use.
High blood pressure or heart disease	Cold, flu, and cough medications that contain sympathomimetics (decongestants), both in oral form and in nasal administration, can increase blood pressure. Antihistamines (in large doses) may affect heart rhythm.
Stomach ulcers or persistent heartburn	Aspirin and NSAIDs can worsen symptoms or even cause stomach bleeding, especially at high doses. In addition, if you take antacids for your stomach ulcers, they may interact with multiple drugs and affect their absorption.
Prostate enlargement	Antihistamines (for allergy, cold, itch, sleep) may worsen urinary symptoms.
Glaucoma	Antihistamines (for allergy, cold, itch, sleep) may worsen visual symptoms by further increasing the pressure inside the eye.
Bleeding or clotting disorder	Be careful with aspirin and NSAIDs because they can affect blood clotting.

(continued)

TABLE 9.1 CONTINUED

Conditions	OTC Medications that May Not Be Appropriate
Asthma	People with asthma have higher chance of being allergic to certain NSAIDs. In addition, NSAIDs may worsen asthma symptoms or provoke an asthma attack.
Epilepsy (or treatment with antiepileptic drugs)	Antihistamines (for allergy, cold, itch, sleep) should be avoided because they may increase the risk for seizures in patients with epilepsy. Antiepileptic drugs may have multiple drug interactions and can affect OTC drug efficacy and safety.
Diabetes	Some decongestants can raise blood glucose levels. Diabetic patients are at higher risk for kidney failure; NSAIDs, especially at high doses, may further increase this risk. Some syrups contain high amounts of sugar (sometimes around two thirds of the volume). Chose a sugar-free syrup if you have diabetes.
Thyroid disease (or treatment with thyroid hormones)	OTC antacids (e.g., Tums, Maalox) may decrease the absorption of oral thyroid hormone supplements. Thyroid hormones such as levothyroxine (see Chapter 19) should be taken at least 2 hours before antacids.
HIV (or treatment with antiretroviral [HIV] therapy)	Many medications for treating HIV infection interact with other drugs. If you take an HIV medication "cocktail," you should consult with your physician before taking OTC medications.

It is important to recognize that while prescription drugs need to be proved effective to be approved by regulatory authorities for clinical use, the situation is quite different with CAM products. Complementary medicines, or herbs, may be marketed as supplements as long as they do not cause known damage, without the need for showing effectiveness. And many people around the globe, indeed, regularly use various CAM compounds.

The evidence on safety and effectiveness of CAM typically (but not always) is less rigorous than on prescription medications. It doesn't necessarily mean that CAM compounds don't work, but it means that there is incomplete information on the desired and undesired effects of many of these compounds. Does it mean that I need to stop taking an herbal compound from which I greatly benefit, if it has not been shown effective in a large clinical study? Not necessarily. As we discussed several times now, there is a variability among individuals, and average responses do not always represent what happens to people at the extremes of the response range. If you take a standard dose of vitamin B and you feel more energetic during the day without any side effects, it may be an appropriate routine to keep, even if *vitamin B* has not been shown to improve energy levels in large clinical trials.

The scenario in which the previous principle of "I think it's helpful, I'll keep taking it" does not apply is *disease prevention*. If you are going to take something every day to prevent a future condition, and potentially expose yourself to side effects, you at least want solid evidence that, on average, the intervention has been demonstrated to prevent that condition.

Just remember that along with the potential benefits of CAM, there are significant health risks associated with incorrect intake of herbs, supplements, and vitamins, and I would like to outline some of the important ones in this chapter.

Thousands of CAM products are available, each with its potential beneficial or harmful effects. Most of the concerns are dose-related, which means that consumption of low doses of marketed herbal supplements is not likely to cause harm. However, the higher the dose, the higher the chance of experiencing undesired effects. Table 9.2 provides a (noncomplete) list of CAM products that require special attention in terms of safety, summarizing the main risks and drug interactions. These are examples to give you an idea of potential harms; providing a compelling review of CAM risks and benefits is beyond the scope of this book.

Besides the specific details outlined earlier in this chapter, the following 10 general tips can help you with the *safe use of OTC drugs:*

1. Read the *Drug Facts* label carefully. Do not exceed the dose and the length of treatment recommended on the label.
2. Know your allergies—and make sure you are not allergic to active or inactive ingredients of an OTC product.
3. If you are trying to treat a problem for which you already receive treatment—consult your doctor *before* using an OTC medication.
4. Check with the doctor or pharmacist to be sure the new OTC medicine can be used with your other drugs.
5. Choose a product because the ingredients are appropriate for the condition (don't choose a product simply because its brand name sounds familiar).
6. Choose a product with the fewest appropriate ingredients. Each additional active ingredient may expose you to unnecessary risks. Avoid taking several medicines that have the same active ingredients.
7. Keep a record of all your current OTC medications and supplements. Show this record to your healthcare provider if you have a new condition, are about to undergo surgery, or receive a new treatment.

Herbal Supplement	Main Uses	Potential Harmful Effects
St John's wort (hypericum)	To help with depressive symptoms	1. Can be dangerous when combined with other antidepressants or drugs that increase the effect of the neurotransmitter serotonin (e.g., certain migraine or pain medications) 2. St. John's wort is an inducer of liver CYP enzymes and may interact with many medications by this mechanism (see Chapter 8)
Kava	To alleviate anxiety	May negatively affect liver function, especially when combined with other drugs that may cause liver toxicity
Vitamin A	For treating skin conditions and to prevent eye damage	Long-term high doses increase risk for osteoporosis and bone fractures. Use of large doses in pregnancy may be unsafe for the developing fetus.

(continued)

TABLE 9.2 CONTINUED

Herbal Supplement	Main Uses	Potential Harmful Effects
Vitamin C	To prevent cold or to treat cold and flu symptoms; also for wound healing and various other indications	Daily dietary requirement is about 90 mg/day. Usually safe at doses of 200–1000 mg/day. However, vitamin C in high doses may increase the risk for kidney stones.
Iron	To treat iron-deficiency anemia	It is important not to exceed recommended iron doses. Overdose can be dangerous, especially in children. Many minerals such as calcium, magnesium, and antacids in general interfere with iron absorption. Separate 2 hours from dairy products. Keep away from children.
Gingko	To improve memory and cognitive ability	Gingko, cranberry juice, pomegranate concentrate (or juice), and evening primrose oil increase the chance of *bleeding* when combined with drugs that prevent blood clotting (see Chapter 13).
Cranberry juice, cranberries	To prevent or treat urinary tract infections	

TABLE 9.2 CONTINUED

Herbal Supplement	Main Uses	Potential Harmful Effects
Pomegranate juice, pomegranate concentrate	As an antioxidant— mainly for improving heart and blood vessel function	
Evening primrose oil	For a variety of conditions including arthritis, bone diseases, heart diseases, and pain	
Comfrey, chaparral, pennyroyal (none is approved for marketing as an OTC product, but they are sold in a variety of spice markets and by online vendors)	For variety of indications	Can be toxic to the liver if consumed by mouth (not applied to the skin), especially in large doses

8. Avoid mixing medicines with alcohol.
9. When giving medicine to children, use the correct meas-uring device to make sure they get the right amount.
10. Keep medicines out of reach of children.

DISEASE PREVENTION

An apple a day keeps the doctor away. We all know that healthy routines can keep us healthier and help us live longer. But what exactly is this daily apple? Is it 30 minutes of exercise and literally a serving of fruit, or is it a daily intake of supplemental *calcium, magnesium, iron, vitamins A to E, folic acid, fish oil, antioxidants,* and *coenzyme Q10?* Well, this is a quite a controversial topic with no single answer.

Let's start by looking at multivitamins. Most multivitamin pills do not seem to produce a clear benefit or harm, although there are studies suggesting both. An excellent example of how to inter-pret (and how easy it is to misinterpret) data from clinical studies is the Physicians' Health Study II published in 2012 in the *Journal of American Medical Association,* which suggested that daily multi-vitamin use can modestly reduce the general prevalence of cancer. This was a large research study in male physicians older than 50 years, most of them well-nourished, nonsmoking, and exercising regularly. If you look at the details of the data, it appears that there is no sig-nificant risk reduction in participants who did not have a history of cancer at the time of starting multivitamins.

Neither is there a risk reduction for specific cancers such as pros-tate or colon cancer. The main benefit (about 27% reduction in cancer risk) seems to be in people who had history of cancer at the time of use of multivitamins. So the rational conclusion is that, *in well-nourished and regularly exercising males older than 50 years, particularly those with a history of cancer, the addition of daily vitamins reduces the risk for new or recurrent cancer.* If you belong to this group, then adding daily multivitamins certainly makes sense. The question is: How beneficial are these multivitamins for someone who is smoking, less well-nourished, younger than 50 years, and a female? The answer is that we can say absolutely nothing about such a person based on this study; she might benefit more or might benefit less. We should be referring to other studies that were perhaps designed to answer that question. The problem is that the media is not likely to post a title like the previous conclusion in italics. The marketable title is likely to look like, "daily multivitamin reduces the risk for cancer," despite being only partially correct, or even misleading. Once such a catchy title is out, most people will never bother to look into the study details. One might assume that these are just vitamins, and in the worst case scenario there is simply no benefit and a few dollars were spent. However, such assumptions are inappropriate. Some vitamins, such as *vitamin A* and *vitamin E*, are currently **not** recommended for cancer prevention because studies have shown that they (especially at high doses) may even increase the risk for cancer.

What I want to highlight is that some supplements may help prevent diseases but may also be harmful. When you take a prescription, OTC, or CAM product to treat an existing condition, some side effects may be acceptable if your treatment goals are achieved. On the other hand, when you take a daily drug or supplement to prevent an as-yet nonexisting condition, any toxicity may be unwarranted, unless it is clear that the potential benefit outweighs the risks. But determining that an intervention has a good risk-to-benefit ratio is easier said than done; it is quite a challenging task to judge the evidence on the effectiveness of preventive approaches, even for a trained clinician.

The information would typically come from one of the three sources:

1. The therapy was demonstrated to be effective in large controlled clinical trials.

2. The therapy is suggested to be effective by small uncontrolled studies and observations.

3. The therapy is claimed to be effective by various people (including healthcare professionals) based on anecdotal experience.

Of course, source 1 would be the most reliable and source 3 the least reliable. Before you start using any compound for disease prevention, you need to make sure there is enough information that this approach is **safe**, and the best scenario is when safety data for large controlled clinical studies are available.

The **effectiveness** is another point of discussion. As one could imagine, much more research exists on treating than preventing medical conditions. One of the main reasons for this is related to the differences in resources required to carry out each type of study. Imagine a new compound (a drug, an herb, a vitamin—any compound) you wish to test in *treating* high blood pressure. To get a sense of whether the compound works or not, you may recruit 200 patients with high blood pressure to a study in which half of the study subjects receive the study compound and the other half receive an inactive substance. After 2 months of treatment, you compare the blood pressure parameters of both groups. This 200-patient study might give you at least an idea about whether your intervention is beneficial.

Now imagine that you have a compound that you want to test for *preventing* high blood pressure. In this scenario, you will need to enroll participants with normal blood pressure, treat them with your compound or an inactive substance on a daily basis, and follow up to investigate who among study participants develop high blood pressure. On average, there is about 5% chance for an adult to develop high blood pressure over 2 years. To demonstrate any substantial difference in the rate of high blood pressure development, you might need a 4-year-long study with about 1000 subjects (vs. a 2-month study with 100 subjects being treated and 100 subjects receiving no treatment). You can do the math—you are going to need about 200 times more resources for the prevention study.

Unfortunately, because of the extremely high costs of thorough prevention studies, most data on preventive interventions come from small and uncontrolled studies, which makes them less reliable. This is one of the reasons the recommendations for disease prevention change so often. For example, one day you hear that soy is excellent for your health, the next year it appears that it is not beneficial—and the same goes for certain vitamins, supplements, various diets, and so forth.

If you are thinking about taking CAM treatments for preventing a certain condition, first make sure there is enough information available on the safety of the approach, and second consult a healthcare professional to help with determining whether there is enough evidence to suggest that the approach may be beneficial for your health.

Because of the limitation I described earlier, I am not going to recommend a myriad of preventive routines to improve your health. But I would like to highlight five that are backed up by many years of reliable research and, importantly, common sense.

Routine 1: Exercise Every Week

Physical activity has a countless amount of benefits, and the bottom line is that it prevents premature death. The more you exercise, the lower your risk for dying early. We can pretty safely state that (1) any exercise is better than no exercise, and (2) about 150 minutes of moderate exercise a week (approximately 30 minutes a day, 5 days a week) is where the substantial benefit begins—that amount of exercise can reduce the risk for premature death by roughly 30%. It is recommended that some proportion (between one fourth and one half) of this exercise is vigorous, but if you are unable to perform vigorous activities such as running, walking for half an hour a day is still going to be very beneficial to your health and longevity. The best results in terms of early death prevention are achieved with about 1 hour of exercise every day.

Routine 2: Do Not Smoke

No benefits can be attributed to smoking. And whatever arguments one may have supporting smoking, the hazards of it by far exceed any potential benefit. We have enough research data today showing that exposure (active or passive) to cigarette smoke shortens life. If you smoke and you are between the ages of 25 and 34 years, by quitting now you will gain about 10 extra years of life. If you have been a smoker and you are now between 45 and 59 years, by quitting now you will still gain on average 4 to 5 additional years of life. Of course, quitting is not easy, but there are a variety of pharmacological and psychological approaches that can help. The most important thing is to decide that you want those extra years of life to do things that matter to you, rather than prematurely dying of cancer or a terminal lung disease. Similarly to what we discussed regarding the *why, how,* and *what* questions in Chapter 5, the road to quitting smoking will start with the same question: *Why* is it important that I stop smoking? Once you have convinced yourself that this step is indeed important to you, the rest is going to be technical. Difficult, but doable.

Routine 3: Watch What (and How Much) You Eat

Being overweight increases the risk for many (many!) diseases: high blood pressure, heart disease, arthritis, diabetes, cancer, you name it. A useful measure for estimating whether you are overweight is the body mass index (BMI) rather than your weight in pounds (or kilograms). BMI is calculated as your weight in kilograms (or in pounds divided by 2.2) divided by the square of your height in meters. For example, if you are 6 ft (1.82 m) tall and your weight is 220 lb (100 kg), your BMI will be $100/1.82^2$, that is, $100/3.31 = 30.2$ kg/m^2. Normal BMI ranges between 18.5 and 25; a person with BMI above 25 but below 30 is considered overweight (beside few exceptions like bodybuilders), and someone with BMI above 30 is considered obese.

There is an endless amount of dietary advice available from all over the globe, starting with Mediterranean, fat-free, carbohydrate-free, paleo, gluten-free, or vegetarian diets, through calorie counting and point counting, to individual versus group coaching—you name it. I am not for or against a particular diet, and I am not going to argue about the benefits of any of them. However, I would suggest following these two common sense rules:

Rule 1: You should not put into your body more calories than you burn. And **no**—you should not eat huge amounts of food this week and promise that you will burn all these calories next week.

Rule 2: Whatever diet you choose, it should be balanced with intake of vitamins, protein, and fiber. And **yes**—a little fat and carbohydrates are fine, as long as you follow rule 1.

Starting with Greek philosophers of 5th-century BCE claiming that "nothing comes from nothing," through the establishment of the *principle of mass conservation* outlined in the 18th century, it is clear that you will continue to gain weight as long as you consume more calories than you burn. It is THAT simple. Yes, different people have different metabolism rates, but people who claim that they eat "almost nothing" but keep gaining weight might need to revise their "almost." As an 83-year old Judo master once told me, "One should have the right to consume food not because one can buy it, but because one has earned it by exercising." If you are overweight or obese, there is no way around it: it is only by *eating less* and *exercising more* that you are going to lose weight over time. No tricks, no shortcuts. Even the bariatric (sleeve) surgery is largely aimed at reducing the amount of food you are able to take in. The moment you tip the balance toward more calories burned than gained, you will start losing weight. It may be a slow and difficult process, but you must persevere if you want your results and your health on the right track.

Routine 4: Folic Acid in Pregnancy

If you are a woman of childbearing age and plan to become pregnant or are thinking about that possibility sometime in the near future, take folic acid supplements. A once-a-day folic acid dose between 0.4 and 1mg will do the job, and you might need up to 5 mg if you have certain risk factors. As I will outline in Chapter 10, there is a baseline risk for birth defects of unknown reason. Folic acid is essential for the development of the nervous system and other systems of the fetus—daily intake starting before pregnancy and continuing at least until the end of 12th week of pregnancy can prevent birth defects in the newborn.

Routine 5: Moderation in Alcohol Consumption

Alcohol consumption is related to a large number of potentially serious consequences. However, it is not as straightforward as smoking because some studies have demonstrated that mild consumption of alcohol, especially red wine, may have benefits to your health. But because alcohol is so popular, many do not pay enough attention to their alcohol-consuming habits. And the reality is that long-term alcohol consumption consequences can be negative, and sometimes devastating. Moderate to high consumption of alcoholic drinks increases the risk for several cancers, including of breast, head and neck, stomach, liver, and colon. Long-lasting alcohol use may cause serious liver disease, impairment in cognitive ability, and other problems such as pancreatitis and nerve damage leading to persistent loss of sensation and pain in the feet. In addition, chronic alcohol use can cause liver CYP enzyme induction and reduce the effectiveness of some of your drugs. An occasional social drink may not bear much harm (given you are neither driving nor pregnant), but avoid making alcohol consumption a habit—there are too many negative consequences associated with it.

Take-Home Message

Although most of us have a trusted healthcare professional we can consult with, there will be many situations in which you will need to be making your own decisions about your health, your diseases and their treatment, and prevention of future diseases. One of these situations is the use of OTC and CAM products. You should be aware of what kind of OTC drugs and supplements are not appropriate for you, and you should consult with a pharmacist or a physician before using these if you have a chronic condition or you are taking drugs on a constant basis.

Lifestyle habits for preventing diseases are at least as important, and here too, many decisions are to be made by you. Avoiding smoking, limiting your alcohol consumption, maintaining a normal BMI, eating in moderation, and engaging in physical activity on a regular basis are all evidence-based approaches that in combination can both prolong your life and improve its quality.

[10]

DRUGS IN PREGNANCY
AND BREASTFEEDING

PREGNANCY

You wake up with a headache. It's that familiar old pain you have from time to time. Almost on an autopilot, you reach out to the bottle of painkillers you always have in your bedside table drawer, and one moment before taking a pill you remember—"Oh, wait a minute, I am 6 weeks pregnant!" Your head is now really splitting, but should you take that pain killer?

A pregnant woman, on average, takes between two and 15 different medications during her pregnancy for treating nausea, pain, swelling, common cold, and other conditions. Although everything we have previously discussed regarding drug safety and effectiveness applies to pregnant women as well, there are two **additional** important issues to consider when taking drugs during pregnancy. The first issue is that the medication may cross the placenta and affect the developing baby (the *fetus*). The second issue is that the body of a pregnant woman undergoes substantial changes that can affect drug pharmacokinetics and also pharmacodynamics.

Drug Effects on the Developing Fetus

Let's look first at the potential effects on the developing baby, which is the more critical issue. On average, 3 to 6% of all newborns suffer from some kind of birth defect (or birth abnormality). These vary from cognitive deficits, growth retardation, and cosmetic defects such as minor cleft lip, through serious heart defects that require surgical intervention, to conditions such as trisomy 21 (Down syndrome) that currently are neither preventable nor treatable. In most of these cases, there is no clear, identifiable cause that has led to the condition. Some drugs that I will discuss in this chapter have been associated with increased risks for such defects, although it is very important to state that because of the baseline risk, it is difficult to determine how much additional risk a certain drug adds to an individual woman. If the pregnant woman has certain medical conditions such as diabetes, this baseline risk increases even further, making it challenging to determine the safety of drugs on the developing baby.

Since it is not feasible and not ethical to perform clinical trials in pregnant women just for the sake of testing whether a drug is safe in pregnancy or not, most of the available information on how drugs affect a developing baby comes from case reports in the literature. Large databases such as Reprotox collect information from these case reports and various population studies looking at associations between drug exposure and pregnancy outcomes, and provide summaries on currently available information regarding the potentially harmful effects of specific drugs in pregnancy. By comparing whether women who were exposed to a certain drug in pregnancy have different outcomes compared with similar women who were not exposed to that drug, more reliable data can be generated. The information available from animal experiments can sometimes be helpful in clarifying the risk, although the "translation" of pregnant mouse studies to humans is usually not straightforward and needs to be interpreted with caution.

Given the baseline 3 to 6% risk for birth defects, it is also difficult to truly determine the usefulness of single case reports. Let's look at an example, just to get a sense of the challenge in correctly assigning the likelihood of an undesirable outcome to drug exposure.

Julia is a 34-year-old woman in the third month of pregnancy with her second child. She had been suffering from anxiety attacks once in a while before pregnancy, and she has an anxiolytic (antianxiety) medication that she has been taking on and off. This time, the anxiety attacks are quite bad, and she really struggles with the decision of whether to take her medicine. She eventually decides to take it for a few days, and the treatment really helps with her symptoms. The rest of Julia's pregnancy is uneventful, but the baby is born with a cleft palate.

What is the likelihood that a few days' treatment with the anxiolytic drug has caused, or contributed to, the cleft palate defect in Julia's child? Statistically, one of every 900 children is born with a cleft palate. Could this be simply a coincidence and the baby would have been born with the birth defect anyway? As you can imagine, the question is quite hard to answer in retrospect. As we discussed in Chapter 2, it is important to differentiate between association and causality. As long as causality (i.e., drug X has caused the defect Y) has not been established, it's unjustified to "blame" the drug. One could also blame Julia's coffee consumption, an alcohol drinking episode in the fourth week of her pregnancy (when she didn't know she was pregnant), or genetics, since one of her husband's nephews was also born with a cleft palate.

You get the idea—when a child is born with a defect, it is very challenging to point to one specific factor (e.g., a drug) responsible for it. On the other hand, the information collected over the decades indicates that certain drugs are associated with certain birth abnormalities. For example, alcohol consumption during pregnancy is associated with a very specific set of abnormalities called *fetal alcohol syndrome*. *Warfarin* (for clotting disorders; see Chapter 13) is associated with *fetal warfarin syndrome*. By collecting all the available information from research studies, case reports, and animal experiments, the regulatory agencies such as the US Food and Drug Administration (FDA) assign pregnancy risk category to each approved drug (and the category assignment is updated when more information is available). These categories are named A, B, C, D, and X.

Category A drugs are considered safe in pregnancy. Unfortunately, there are very few drugs in this category. *Category B* drugs are often used in pregnancy because animal studies do not suggest added risk, but as opposed to category A, reliable human studies supporting safe use in pregnancy are lacking. *Category C* is quite confusing. Many drugs are classified in this category. For drugs in this class, usually some harm has been demonstrated in animal studies, or certain case reports in humans reported, but the causality is not clear. These are the most difficult drugs to decide on, and the decision of whether to use them or not is determined on an individual basis. For *category D* drugs, some evidence of fetal risk has been demonstrated, and thorough consideration needs to be given to whether the therapeutic effect can outweigh the risks. Many of drugs in this category are drugs for treating seizure disorders. They can increase the risk for nervous system disorders in the fetus, but on the other hand, if an epileptic mother is not treated and has a seizure, it may substantially increase the risk for the developing fetus. Therefore, the decision to use category D drugs will be made on an individual basis, after you and your physician carefully consider your risks and the potential benefits. *Category X* drugs are known to cause substantial increase in risk for birth defects and must be avoided in pregnancy and in women who may become pregnant. For example, *isotretinoin* (for treating acne), *warfarin* (for treating clotting disorders), certain *hormones*, and many *anticancer chemotherapy drugs* belong to this category.

Typically, the most critical period of the baby's organ formation (*organogenesis*) is the first 12 weeks of pregnancy. This is the time window when the developing fetus is the most vulnerable to toxic effects that could result in structural abnormalities. Beyond the 12th week of pregnancy, if any toxic effects occur, they would be primarily affecting the baby's development and cognition. As a general rule, drugs should be avoided in pregnancy unless there is a clear need for taking the drug and the benefit outweighs the potential risk to the developing baby.

One point I would like to make is regarding various *natural* or *herbal* supplements, or complementary and alternative medicine (CAM). The thought may be that since these are natural, they are safe in pregnancy. This is certainly not the case. While many drugs are systematically studied and their risks are known, we do not know what most herbal supplements do or how they can affect the developing baby. I would suggest refraining from using CAM products in pregnancy, unless there are reliable data to support their safety.

Pharmacokinetic and Pharmacodynamic Changes during Pregnancy

The effect of some drugs may change during pregnancy, especially during the last term (trimester). Naturally, women gain weight during pregnancy, and sometimes this gain is quite substantial—around 35 to 40 lb (or 15 to 20 kg). If we try to think in percent change, as we frequently did in previous chapters referring to drug exposure, for women who were overweight before pregnancy this can be a 20 to 25% change, but for women who were underweight before pregnancy, this can be a 30 to 40% increase in weight. As a result of this gain in weight and an increase in the amount of plasma (blood fluids) in pregnancy, the concentration of some drugs in the blood can be substantially reduced if the standard dosing is continued. This may be relevant to thyroid hormones, antiepileptic drugs, and certain antibiotics. Passage of fluids through the kidneys is enhanced during pregnancy; therefore, some drugs that are cleared by the kidney may be excreted faster. Given these changes, if you are taking chronic drugs and become pregnant, it is always useful to consult your obstetrician about any changes that may be necessary in drugs or drug doses during pregnancy, even if the drug itself is considered safe.

BREASTFEEDING

Breastfeeding is one of the most natural acts in mammals, including humans. There are numerous potential benefits of breastfeeding, and indeed, the majority of the world's babies are breastfed. On the other hand, with the highly scientific approach to manufacturing of baby formulas, millions of healthy babies worldwide grow up without receiving breast milk. The discussion of whether to breastfeed is well beyond the scope of this book, and it should be an individual decision that the parents make (or have to make) based on circumstances and their beliefs. What I want to present in this chapter are a few rules of thumb about taking medications, if you decided to breastfeed.

Between 90 and 99% of women who are breastfeeding will receive at least one medication during that period, especially in the first few weeks after delivery. When a nursing mother takes a drug that is intended to work systemically, some portion of it will be distributed into the breast milk. The extent of this distribution will depend on the physical, chemical, and pharmacokinetic properties of the drug. That portion can be tiny and insignificant for some drugs but substantial for others.

One of the most common situations (which require treatment) that mothers encounter is pain after delivery. The most frequent causes are surgical pain after a cesarean delivery or episiotomy (a surgical incision of the perineum during labor). It is important to relieve the mother's pain in order for her to take a proper care of her child(ren). On the other hand, it is important to understand what are the drugs (and their doses) that are safe during this period.

In the immediate period after the birth, while at the hospital, you might be treated with a variety of approaches, including epidural analgesia for the first couple of days if you underwent a cesarean delivery. You may also be given drugs intravenously or orally to help with the pain. Drugs such as *acetaminophen* (*paracetamol*) and nonsteroidal anti-inflammatory drugs (NSAIDs) such as *ibuprofen* are considered safe during breastfeeding. In case the pain is substantial and these painkillers are not effective, stronger pain relief medications can be considered, such as *morphine* or *oxycodone*. These are generally considered compatible with breastfeeding in small doses for a limited use over a few days. As I discussed in Chapter 6 (and will discuss in greater detail in Chapter 18), the most serious adverse effects with morphine-like (opioid) analgesics containing *morphine, oxycodone* (e.g., Percocet), and *hydrocodone* (e.g., Vicodin) are sleepiness and impaired breathing. It is of extreme importance not to exceed the recommended doses of these medications while breastfeeding. If you are in a lot of pain, even high doses of opioid analgesics may not cause serious side effects **to you**. However, since the baby, who gets some of these opioids through breast milk, is not in pain, she is more likely to be affected by side effects such as sleepiness and decreased breathing, if you use excessive doses of these drugs. If you are prescribed one of these drugs during breastfeeding, your doctor will initially monitor for signs of sleepiness, constipation, or reduced breathing in the baby and instruct you to do so later on your own.

Two types of such opioid analgesics that are now *not recommended* during breastfeeding are **codeine** and **tramadol**. Although probably safe in *most* breastfeeding women, these medications can be very dangerous in some. Keep in mind from the discussion in Chapter 3 that some people are *slow metabolizers* of drugs based on their cytochrome P-450 (CYP) enzyme genetics. On the other hand, some people are *ultrarapid metabolizers* and break down drugs faster than an average person. This means that most drugs will not work as well for *ultrarapid metabolizers* because of lower concentrations. However, in the case of *codeine*, the situation is very different. Codeine undergoes metabolism by a CYP enzyme called CYP2D6. In this particular case of codeine, the enzyme does not neutralize the drug but instead turns it into *morphine* (which gives the analgesic effect). In those women who are genetically ultrarapid metabolizers (in whom CYP2D6 works more efficiently), taking codeine will result in a higher than expected concentration of morphine in the blood, which may cause side effects such as sleepiness or nausea. *Morphine* does pass to the breast milk, and in some cases its concentration in breast milk can be so high that the nursing baby absorbs an amount substantial enough to cause side effects. Depending on how small the baby is and on the codeine dose, this amount of *morphine* in an ultrarapid-metabolizing mother's breast milk can be dangerous for the baby. This has resulted in banning codeine administration to breastfeeding mothers, and the use of codeine as analgesic has decreased substantially. The same logic applies to tramadol, which is metabolized by the liver to a more active compound. While these are extreme examples of side effects based on individual differences among patients, healthcare professionals encounter more subtle cases daily and may recommend personalized adjustment of the drug or the dose.

The reality is that there is very little research in this field. It is pretty clear that a mother would not be enthusiastic to participate in research studies in which she is given drugs during breastfeeding and blood samples are taken from her baby to determine how much drug the baby is exposed to. On the other hand, the FDA typically mandates the pharmaceutical companies to have an explicit section in the drug leaflet regarding the safety of the drug during breastfeeding. Databases such as LactMed provide a summary of the available information on the safety of drugs during breastfeeding and can help mothers and clinicians make informed decisions about use of drugs during breastfeeding.

One point to remember is that whatever portion of the drug appeared in the breast milk, the infant takes it by mouth—so the drug may cause systemic side effects *only if it is orally absorbed*. For example, if a mother injects insulin for the treatment of her diabetes, and a proportion of insulin reaches the breast milk, there is no risk that the baby will suffer from a low sugar (glucose) level because of the insulin effect. The reason is that insulin will not be absorbed from the baby's intestines to the blood because it is neutralized in the stomach (otherwise, diabetics could take insulin pills instead of injections). Therefore, the use of insulin by breastfeeding mothers is safe for their baby.

With most drugs, less than 1% of the dose the mother took will eventually get to the nursing baby. To err on the safe side, one could use a rule of thumb and assume that the baby, through breastmilk, may get between 1 and 5% of the drug that the mother took. If that dose, given orally to a baby of that age, is safe, there should not be a reason for particular concern (Table 10.1), except in special cases such as codeine. However, if the drug has not been tested in children, or small doses may have toxic effects, a thorough risk-to-benefit assessment should be performed with your physician, and preferably with your child's pediatrician if the case is for long-term treatment. Let me illustrate how this rule of thumb works (Table 10.1).

TABLE 10.1 APPROXIMATED EXAMPLE OF DRUG PASSAGE
FROM MOTHER TO NURSING BABY THROUGH BREAST MILK

Drug	Daily Oral Dose in Nursing Mother	Approximate Amount in Milk (1–5% of Maternal Dose)	Amount that Can Be Safely Administered Orally to 5-kg Baby
Acetaminophen	3000 mg	30–150 mg/day	200–450 mg/day
Amoxicillin	1500 mg	15–75 mg/day	250–450 mg/day

- *Acetaminophen for pain.* A mother takes 3000 mg/day for her knee pain. Rule of thumb: the baby gets between 1 and 5%, that is, between 30 and 150 mg/day. Let's assume the baby weighs 11 lb (5 kg). The usual dose of acetaminophen in infants is 10 to 15 mg/kg body weight, every 4 to 6 hours (the safe range for this baby, therefore, is 200 to 540 mg/day). Receiving 30 mg/day (and in the worst-case scenario, 150 mg/day) from her mother should probably be safe in this case.
- *Amoxicillin for infection.* The mother takes 500 mg 3 times a day for treating an infection. Rule of thumb: the baby will get between 15 mg (1%) and 75 mg (5%) amoxicillin a day through breast milk. The usual dose of amoxicillin in infants is 50 to 90 mg/kg body weight a day; therefore, the safe range for this 5-kg baby would be 250 to 450 mg/day. Receiving 15 mg (and in the worst-case scenario 75 mg) from her mother should probably be safe in this case.

Indeed, both drugs are compatible with breastfeeding according to the American Academy of Pediatrics.

For many drugs, your doctor will look for the available information on the *blood-to–breast milk ratio* of the drug, which can allow estimating the concentration of the drug in the breast milk. For example, if it is known that a 25-mg dose of *drug A* results in 1 mg/ L concentration in blood, and the blood-to-milk ratio is 1, we assume that the drug concentration in the milk will be about 1 mg/ L as well. Therefore, if the baby drinks five ounces (150 mL) of milk at each feeding, she will receive approximately 0.15 mg of the drug. Assuming she is exclusively breastfed, 5 times a day, the baby will be receiving 0.75 mg of the drug (roughly 3% of the mother's dose). With such numbers available, your doctor could help you make an informed decision on the child's risk associated with breastfeeding while you are taking the medication.

Another example of a substance that reaches a 1:1 ratio between blood and breast milk is *alcohol*. If you drink an alcoholic beverage, the alcohol will appear in your breast milk in about 20 to 30 minutes. As with drugs, the alcohol will not be "stored" in the breast milk but will disappear when it disappears from the blood (remember—1:1 ratio between blood and milk). I want to be clear that drinking alcohol while breastfeeding is generally a bad idea. Drinking on a regular basis, even one drink a day, can reduce the production of breastmilk, cause the baby to eat less, and cause impairment in the child's motor skills. With that said, if you just wish to enjoy an occasional social drink, you probably can if you plan ahead. Three to 4 hours after a single drink, the concentration of alcohol in your blood (and therefore in your breast milk) is going to be very low. You can pump and store milk ahead of time and feed your baby a bottle of the stored (alcohol-free) milk if she needs to eat within 3 to 4 hours from the time you started you drink. Given that you did not have another drink, it should be safe to resume breastfeeding 4 hours after it. Remember that if you had several drinks, it will take longer for the alcohol to get out of your blood (and breast milk).

The primary concern with drugs and breastfeeding is in very little babies, who weigh only a few kilograms. The additional major concern is with particularly toxic drugs, such as those used for cancer chemotherapy, drugs that suppress the immune system, antiepileptic drugs, illicit substances such as *amphetamines* and *heroin*, and several antiarrhythmic drugs such as *amiodarone*.

In some cases, the prescription drug (the safety of which in breastfeeding is not entirely clear) is a medical necessity, and you have to take it. By consulting with your doctor, you may decide not to breastfeed (for the duration of drug intake), but there are also alternatives if you wish to continue breastfeeding. Your doctor can help you decide what would be the optimal time to take the drug in reference to breastfeeding. The answer somewhat depends on the drug's pharmacokinetics. For drugs with a short half-life, it is usually advisable to take them immediately after breastfeeding the baby so that, by the time of the next feeding, a relatively small amount remains in the milk. This practice, however, will change from drug to drug.

Take-Home Message

A few drugs, when taken during pregnancy, may cause defects or abnormalities in the developing baby. In general, drugs (and especially alcohol and cigarette smoking) should be avoided during pregnancy. However, some drugs can be used safely in pregnancy, and in many cases the use of the drug (for the mother's health) is important enough to outweigh the potential risks to the baby. In all cases, consult with your physician in advance about the appropriateness of drug use during pregnancy. The general approach is similar for taking drugs if you are breastfeeding. The goal should be to prevent unnecessary exposure of the infant to drugs. With that said, many drugs are safe in breastfeeding, and your physician can help you decide on the circumstances in which the risk to the infant is small enough to justify taking the drug.

PART II

MEDICATION THERAPY TIPS IN COMMON DISEASE STATES

In the second half of the book, I will illustrate how one can use the information acquired by reading Chapters 1 to 10 for the treatment of specific conditions. The information in Part I was rather general, and this is the opportunity to examine how it can be applied to the real-life setting. The chapters of Part II focus on 10 common conditions that typically require treatment with drugs, although there are certainly many more important conditions for which drug knowledge is required for safe, effective, and responsible treatment at home. The structures of the chapters are relatively uniform to make it easier to follow, but each chapter has a somewhat different length and focus, as the treatment approach in each condition is often unique. For some conditions, such as high blood pressure, most of the drugs are relatively safe; therefore, the focus is on the overall approach to achieving the treatment goals. In other conditions, such as seizure disorders, the drugs are very complex and have multiple safety issues; therefore, the chapter is more heavily focused on the individual differences among drugs, their side effects, and drug interactions. By learning from these examples, I am hoping that you will be able to apply these principles to your individual conditions and medications. This way, together with your trusted healthcare professionals, you will be able to attain the optimal goals of your treatment.

Please note that each chapter provides an outlook on a single condition. Your other conditions, or the other drugs you take, may affect the treatment you eventually receive. In addition, the chapters are not a guideline for treating diseases but instead are a general overview of each condition, treatment goals, and the common drugs available for treating the disorder. As you will notice, the description of the relevant drugs, whether appearing in a table or as text, is not going to be a comprehensive professional-level review. Neither will it supply **all** the information required for safe and effective treatment of your condition. Remember: the information in this book is not a medical advice, and it is not intended to replace the recommendations and advice of your physician. The goal is to provide you with the key elements of treatment approach and available drugs as well as the desired outcomes and tools for the assessment of treatment success. For you, the optimal treatment will be determined by a clinician who knows you and your medical history. By reading the relevant chapters, however, you will be able to understand the treatment principles and ask important questions to improve your outcomes.

When I mention specific drugs, I will provide the generic name of the drug and give an example or two of its common trade names. These examples are not to suggest that any one commercial product is better than another, or that I recommend it. Rather, it simply would not be feasible to mention all trade names for each product.

To summarize, Part II of this book is not a guide for self-treatment of the described conditions; it is a resource to help you to understand better the goals of your pharmacological treatment as they relate to your conditions and to ask the right questions for achieving those goals in an effective and safe manner.

[11]

HIGH BLOOD PRESSURE

The Silent Killer You Can Stop

High blood pressure, or *hypertension*, is one of the most prevalent chronic disorders and is a common reason for the use of prescription drugs. Approximately 30% of adults in the United States are affected by high blood pressure. In fact, high blood pressure has become so common that some people are not even making a "big deal" of it and do not consider it a serious disease. This is absurd, honestly, because hypertension is one of the main contributors to heart attacks, strokes, and kidney diseases. So let's be very clear about this: high blood pressure is a disease, and quite a dangerous one.

Hypertension is usually diagnosed based on two or more high blood pressure measurements of above 140/90 mm Hg. Ideally, your blood pressure levels should be around 120/80 mm Hg. The first (higher) number is termed *systolic blood pressure* (this is the pressure in the blood vessels when the heart contracts), and the second, lower, number is termed *diastolic blood pressure* and reflects the pressure of the blood when the heart is resting between each two beats. High blood pressure can appear without any apparent cause or can have a known cause such as kidney disease or a long-term use of certain drugs such as *corticosteroids*, decongestants like *pseudoephedrine*, and illicit substances such as *methamphetamine* and *cocaine*. The risk for high blood pressure increases with age, weight gain, excessive alcohol consumption, lack of physical activity, and presence of diabetes and high blood cholesterol. It is also affected by race and is more prevalent and severe in African Americans.

High blood pressure is a tricky condition, and as I already mentioned, it is dangerous. Uncontrolled hypertension causes damage to the blood vessels in the heart and the brain, which can result in a heart attack or stroke as well as damage small blood vessels (capillaries) in the eyes and the kidneys. Unfortunately, it is difficult to diagnose hypertension early because people frequently do not have any symptoms until some damage has already occurred. You may suffer from tiredness or headaches as symptoms of high blood pressure, but the symptoms are very nonspecific and are common to many other conditions. In fact, hypertension is usually diagnosed accidentally, either during a routine checkup in the physician's office or during an emergency department or hospital visit. After hypertension is diagnosed, however, it is very important to make your best effort to keep the blood pressure under control. Extensive research performed in the past several decades has clearly shown that good control of blood pressure reduces the risk of heart failure by half, the risk for stroke by one third, and the risk for heart attack by about one fourth.

TREATMENT GOALS

The ultimate goal of treating high blood pressure is to prevent damage to the heart, the brain, and the kidneys. But as I have previously mentioned, it is difficult to measure your success along the way when you are trying to *prevent* a condition. Fortunately, the blood pressure measurement *itself* acts as a decent surrogate of treatment success. Therefore, the aim should be to control your blood pressure according to the goals recommended by your physician. It's important to understand that the precise blood pressure goal may vary a bit among individuals.

Although blood pressure below 130/85 mm Hg would be an ideal goal for most adults, for people with certain conditions less aggressive goals might be more appropriate. It is not necessary to control high blood pressure only with drugs. Some people are able to reduce or even normalize their blood pressure with diet and regular exercise. This should be the first step in any person diagnosed with high blood pressure. The minimum nondrug modalities should include restriction of salt in the diet, limitation of alcohol intake, weight loss in overweight and obese patients, and regular aerobic exercise regardless of weight. Every patient diagnosed with hypertension should make the maximum effort to make these changes. By skipping those and "jumping" directly to medications you are depriving yourself of a good chance to make a long-term contribution to your health. The routines I outlined in Chapter 9 (being physically active, not smoking, controlling your weight, and limiting alcohol) would be an appropriate starting point for these lifestyle modifications. Even if they are not entirely effective in controlling your blood pressure, by maintaining a diet and exercise routine and close-to-normal weight, your blood pressure medications will have a higher chance to be effective if you start treatment. You are then also likely to need fewer medications with lower doses, which will reduce the chance of experiencing undesired side effects.

TREATMENT APPROACH

After you and your physician have reached the conclusion that you need to start drug treatment for hypertension, the immediate goal will be to control or normalize your blood pressure. You may need only one drug to control high blood pressure, but more commonly, a combination of drugs may be needed. It is worth noting that the important thing in hypertension is achieving the blood pressure goals rather than receiving a certain combination of medications.

Several groups of medications exist for treating high blood pressure. Most of these reduce the blood pressure by decreasing the resistance of small blood vessels and/or by slowing down the heart rate so that there is less pressure against which the blood flows in the blood vessels. Table 11.1 summarizes the major drug classes available for managing hypertension, with a general description of how they work, highlighting some of the most important side effects and special instructions that you should be aware of.

SPECIFIC DRUGS
Thiazide Diuretics

Thiazide diuretic drugs reduce blood pressure by moving fluid (water) from blood to the urine through the kidneys. As their name implies, they will cause diuresis, which means increased urination. It is usually recommended not to take these medications before going to sleep so that you won't need to wake up at night to use the bathroom. Most of these medications, for example *hydrochlorothiazide* (sometimes abbreviated as *HCTZ*), are taken once daily, in the morning.

Diuretics may cause electrolyte (salt) imbalance in the body. Some may cause the level of electrolytes, such as sodium, calcium, magnesium, or potassium, to increase or decrease in the blood. If you are prescribed a diuretic, your doctor will monitor your electrolytes from time to time by ordering some blood tests, approximately twice a year. If not, it might be a good idea to remind your doctor to do this.

TABLE 11.1 COMMON DRUG FOR THE TREATMENT OF HIGH BLOOD PRESSURE

Drug Class and Example(s)	Mechanism of Action	Most Common and Unique Side Effects	Special Instructions and Tips
Thiazide diuretics Hydrochlorothiazide, or HCTZ (Microzide, others) Indapamide (Lozol) Chlorthalidone (Thalitone)	Reduce blood pressure by moving fluid (water) from blood to the urine through the kidneys	Dizziness and lightheadedness on standing up from sitting/ lying position Blood electrolyte (salt) imbalances	Usually taken once a day in the morning Blood tests for electrolyte levels are recommended periodically
ACE inhibitors Lisinopril (Prinivil, others) Enalapril (Vasotec, others) Ramipril (Altace, others) Captopril (Capoten, others) Fosinopril (Monopril)	Angiotensin-converting enzyme (ACE) enables the production of angiotensin II, a molecule that narrows blood vessels and can increase blood pressure. By inhibiting ACE, these drugs reduce the amount of angiotensin II and prevent the increase in blood pressure	Dry cough Elevated blood potassium levels (hyperkalemia) **Rare**: angioedema— swelling of tissues such as the tongue and the lips	Not to be used in pregnancy Blood tests for potassium levels are recommended periodically

(*continued*)

TABLE 11.1 CONTINUED

Drug Class and Example(s)	Mechanism of Action	Most Common and Unique Side Effects	Special Instructions and Tips
Angiotensin II receptor blockers (ARBs) Losartan (Cozaar) Candesartan (Atacand)	ARBs block the effects of angiotensin II on blood vessels and prevent blood vessel narrowing		
Calcium channel blockers			
1. Dihydropyridine calcium channel blockers Amlodipine (Norvasc) Felodipine (Plendil)	By blocking calcium channels within the smooth muscle cells of blood vessels, these drugs prevent blood vessel narrowing. This eventually reduces blood vessel resistance and decreases blood pressure	Swelling of the limbs, palpitations, increased heart rate Flushing	Refrain from grapefruit juice while taking drugs from this group (particularly felodipine)

2. Nondihydropyridine calcium channel blockers Diltiazem (Cardizem, others) Verapamil (Calan, Covera-HS, others)	These drugs block calcium channels as described for dihydropyridines but also do so in the muscle cells in the heart. This activity reduces the strength and frequency of heart contractions and further contributes to reduction in blood pressure	Slow heart rate Constipation	Be aware that both verapamil and diltiazem have many potential drug–drug interactions
Beta-blockers Atenolol (Tenormin, others) Metoprolol (Lopressor, others) Bisoprolol (Zebeta, others)	These drugs block beta-1 and/or beta-2 receptors. Like nondihydropyridine calcium channel blockers, beta-blockers slow heart rate and reduce heart contraction force but also reduce the resistance of blood vessels	Slow heart rate Tiredness Headache	Some beta-blockers (e.g., propranolol) are not appropriate for patients with asthma. Diabetic patients need to be aware that beta-blockers may "mask" some of the symptoms of hypoglycemia (fall in blood glucose level)

Angiotensin-Converting Enzyme Inhibitors

Angiotensin-converting enzyme (ACE) mediates the production of angiotensin II, a molecule that binds to a receptor called (unsurprisingly) the angiotensin II receptor in blood vessels and causes a constriction of the vessels, which causes an increase in blood pressure. ACE inhibitors reduce the amount of produced angiotensin II, thus causing less reduction in blood vessel diameter and promoting a decrease in blood pressure.

Most patients with high blood pressure, unless they have a contraindication (a condition in which the drug should not be prescribed), will be prescribed an ACE inhibitor. There are several drugs in the group, their names ending with *pril*—*enalapril, ramipril, captopril, lisinopril,* and others. Most of them are prescribed once or twice a day. One of the common side effects associated with ACE inhibitors is dry cough. It happens in about one of every 10 to 20 people, will typically start a few weeks after treatment initiation, and is more common in the Chinese population. When the ACE inhibitor is discontinued, the cough will typically go away. There is little value in switching the treatment to another ACE inhibitor because there is a high chance that the cough will be back. In most cases, it's a better idea to try treatment with another group of drugs if the dry cough becomes inconvenient and cannot be tolerated.

Another common side effect associated with ACE inhibitor use is dizziness, which can be minimized by starting at a low dose. Increase in blood potassium (hyperkalemia) is another somewhat frequent side effect that occurs in about one of 30 patients treated with ACE inhibitors. Be sure your doctor orders periodic measurement of blood potassium levels if you are treated with an ACE inhibitor.

One somewhat confusing complication of ACE inhibitor treatment is the worsening of kidney function in patients with certain preexisting kidney conditions. On one hand, ACE inhibitors can *prevent* kidney damage in patients with diabetes, but on the other hand, they can *worsen* kidney function in other kidney diseases. Always consult your doctor about the appropriateness of ACE inhibitors if you have any kidney condition.

Lastly, a rare but potentially dangerous side effect is *angioedema*, a swelling of the lips, tongue, or face. Because it might not be possible to prevent this condition, it is important to be educated about it and to immediately seek medical care if any of these swelling symptoms occur. The symptoms may be immediate after starting the drug or delayed by several months. ACE inhibitors should be avoided in pregnancy because their use in pregnancy may cause malformations in the developing baby.

Angiotensin Receptor Blockers

Angiotensin receptor blockers (ARBs) work by a mechanism that is similar to ACE inhibitors, but instead of blocking the production of angiotensin II, they prevent (block) the binding of angiotensin II to its receptor on blood vessels so that angiotensin II cannot cause an increase in blood pressure.

The names of the drugs in this group end with *sartan*, for example, *losartan, candesartan*, and *olmesartan*. ARBs are usually taken once a day, and their side effects and monitoring requirements are similar to those of ACE inhibitors. As with ACE inhibitors, they should be avoided in pregnancy.

Calcium Channel Blockers

Calcium within the smooth muscle cells of blood vessels is required for contraction of these muscles, which narrows the blood vessel. By blocking calcium channels, these drugs prevent smooth muscle contraction and prevent the narrowing of blood vessels. This eventually reduces the resistance of blood vessels and decreases the blood pressure.

Calcium has a similar role in the heart muscle because it promotes heart muscle contractions (heartbeat) and can affect the rate and the force of the contraction. Higher rate and higher force of heart muscle contraction will pump more blood into the blood vessels and will result in an increase in the blood pressure. Therefore, if calcium channels in the heart muscle are blocked, the reduction of heartbeat frequency and force will result in decrease of blood pressure.

There are several subgroups of drugs that belong to the group of calcium channel blockers. The ones more often prescribed for treating high blood pressure are called "dihydropyridines," and most of their names end with *dipine: nifedipine, felodipine,* and *amlodipine.* They block mainly calcium channels on the blood vessels, not in the heart, and reduce their resistance. Their duration of action is usually long enough to be taken once a day. Previously used short-acting oral or sublingual (under the tongue) formulations of the calcium channel blocker *nifedipine* were found to be associated with serious side effects and are rarely used for treating hypertension today.

There are other types of calcium channel blockers, which are collectively called nondihydropyridines. The main representatives of this group are *verapamil* (e.g., Calan, Isoptin) and *diltiazem* (e.g., Cardizem). Beyond acting on peripheral vessels, these drugs block the calcium channels in the heart and decrease heart rate and contraction force.

The *side effects* associated with dihydropyridine calcium channel blockers are somewhat different from the nondihydropyridine ones. Among common side effects of *dihydropyridines* calcium channel blockers are headaches, flushing (redness and warmth of the skin, mainly in the face), and swelling of the extremities (called *edema*)— all resulting from excessive widening of blood vessels. The side effects associated with *nondihydropyridines* may include changes in heart rhythm (primarily decreased heart rate), constipation, and thickening of the gums. Both *verapamil* and *diltiazem* are also prone to interactions with other drugs. They are strong inhibitors of liver CYP enzymes and can inhibit the metabolism of many other drugs, resulting in increased side effects of the "affected" drug. If you take *verapamil* or *diltiazem*, consult with your doctor or the pharmacist every time you take an additional prescription or over-the-counter drug. In addition, these calcium channel blockers might slow the heart rate too much if combined with other drugs that decrease heart rate, for example, beta-blockers. It is important to know that some calcium channel blockers (e.g., *felodipine*) can be affected by drinking grapefruit juice (see Chapter 7).

Beta-Blockers

There are two types of beta receptors (also called beta-adrenergic receptors) relevant to the heart function and blood pressure: beta-1 receptors are located mainly in the heart and promote increased heart rate and contraction force; and beta-2 receptors are located mainly in blood vessels, and their activation promotes constriction (narrowing) of blood vessels. Beta receptors are the targets on which adrenaline (epinephrine) and noradrenaline (norepinephrine) hormones in the body work (see Chapter 4). Some beta-blocker drugs such as *atenolol* are selective to beta-1 receptors, which mean that they block beta-1 receptors at usual doses, without significantly affecting beta-2 receptors. Other beta-blocker drugs, such as *propranolol*, are not selective, which means that at usual doses, they block both beta-1 and beta-2 receptors. Depending on the individual person's needs and existing conditions, the optimal beta-blocker can be chosen among several available ones.

Beta-blockers have historically been among the most frequently used medications for hypertension. Their names end with *olol: propranolol, metoprolol, bisoprolol,* and so forth. Not all beta-blockers are the same; quite important differences exist among them, especially in terms of side effects. Almost all beta-blockers can reduce the heart rate, but they do so to a different extent. Some may cause headache or sexual dysfunction, or worsen depression. Often your physician can help address specific beta-blocker side effects by switching to a different beta-blocker with a different side-effect profile.

Nonselective beta-blockers can worsen asthma because beta-2 receptors are also present in airways (see Chapter 15), and blocking them can cause narrowing of the airways. In general, beta-blockers are not advised in people with asthma, but if treatment is necessary, your doctor can help you make the appropriate choice by prescribing a beta-1 selective drug.

If you have diabetes and are prescribed a beta-blocker, you need to be extra cautious. Beta-blockers may alter carbohydrate metabolism by affecting the release of glucose from the liver and the secretion of insulin from the pancreas. In addition, when glucose levels in the blood drop, one of the usual warning signs is increased heart rate. When you are treated with a beta-blocker, the drug can prevent the increased heartbeats and may "mask" the warning signs of dropped blood sugar. You should then pay more attention to other hypoglycemia signs, such as cold sweats, or consider another treatment for your high blood pressure. Your doctor may recommend a nonselective beta-blockers such as *carvedilol* or *nebivolol,* that have additional mechanisms of action, and might be more appropriate if you have both diabetes and high blood pressure that requires beta-blocker treatment.

Most important, treatment with beta-blockers should *not* be discontinued abruptly. After you have been taking a beta-blocker for more than a few weeks, if it is discontinued at once, you may experience "withdrawal" effects, such as sudden increase in heart rate, chest pain, and even a heart attack if you have an existing heart disease. Therefore, if you need to stop the treatment, your doctor will guide you how to do it gradually.

Patients should be aware of the drug interactions with beta-blockers. Other medications that can reduce the heart rate (e.g., *verapamil* or *diltiazem*, discussed earlier) or cause heart rhythm changes (e.g., a variety of psychiatric medications) should be avoided or used with caution along with frequent heart rhythm monitoring.

Additional Drugs

There are additional drugs used for treating hypertension. Some of them are reserved for more resistant high blood pressure or for special populations such as pregnant women. These include, for example, *methyldopa* (Aldomet) and *clonidine* (Catapres), which work by reducing the overall release of adrenaline and noradrenaline hormones. Another group of drugs are called alpha-blockers, and these drugs include *doxazosin* (Cardura) and *prazosin* (Minipress), although these are not as common for treating hypertension as in that past because newer and safer drugs, like ACE inhibitors and dihydropyridine calcium channel blockers are now available.

Spironolactone (Aldactone) and *eplerenone* (Inspra) are called aldosterone antagonists, and they can help decrease blood pressure by blocking the effect of the hormone aldosterone, which can lead to salt and fluid retention and high blood pressure. Newer drugs such as *aliskiren* (Tekturna) inhibit the production of renin, a protein produced by your kidneys that participates in the production of angiotensin II. One or more of these drugs can be considered by your physician based on your individual response to treatment or other existing conditions.

Combination Pills

Several combination products are available for treating hypertension. They can contain both a diuretic and an ACE inhibitor (e.g., *hydro-chlorothiazide + benazepril*: Lotensin HCT), an ACE inhibitor with a calcium channel blocker (e.g., *benazepril + amlodipine*: Lotrel), or an ARB with a calcium channel blocker (e.g., *valsartan + amlodipine*: Exforge). These are mainly intended to improve the convenience of drug intake for individuals whose blood pressure is controlled by the combination of the medications so that they can take one pill instead of two (or sometimes three).

DRUG-RELATED SPECIAL ISSUES

Don't miss your blood pressure medications! I mentioned that hypertension is a tricky disease because you may not have immediate symptoms, but as long as your blood pressure is high, it causes harm whether you feel it or not. With other conditions that have continuous symptoms, like arthritis, if you forgot to take your analgesic pill, the pain is likely to increase, which will remind you to take your medicine. With hypertension, you may experience no symptoms and assume that the situation is under control. Big mistake. Remember: blood pressure medications work and prevent mortality only if you take them regularly. Some people will wait until they have terrible symptoms (and then the blood pressure will typically be very high), then only take their medication for a few days until the symptoms are gone. This is quite a poor strategy in the long run.

When you begin therapy with any blood pressure medication, avoid standing up rapidly from sitting or lying down, especially in the first week; you may experience a sudden fall in blood pressure and may faint. Allow your body to get used to the new medication(s).

With any new medication, or an increase in the dose of an existing medication, it is usually reasonable to allow a month of treatment to determine whether the blood pressure is well controlled. If by the end of 4 weeks the blood pressure is higher than the determined target, your physician may increase your drug dose or add an additional drug to your regimen.

The drugs mentioned in this chapter are not exclusively used for treating high blood pressure. Many of them are effective in a variety of heart conditions or after a heart attack. If in addition to high blood pressure you have other conditions, the preferred therapy may change, and your physician may prescribe a drug that is optimal for treating both conditions.

SPECIAL POPULATIONS

Many of the blood pressure mediations are dangerous, or not recommended, in pregnancy. ACE inhibitors, for example, the most commonly used medications in nonpregnant adults, are not considered safe in pregnant women. If you are pregnant or plan to become pregnant, consult with your doctor so that you can switch to a safer medication and find the appropriate dose before you become pregnant. Your doctor may recommend *methyldopa, nifedipine, labetalol,* or another medication during pregnancy.

There are data showing that people of African ancestry have better treatment outcomes with thiazide diuretics or calcium channel blockers than with ACE inhibitors. Therefore, if you are, for example, African American, these two groups of drugs may be the preferred initial choice for treating your high blood pressure.

IMPORTANT QUESTIONS TO ASK YOUR DOCTOR

- Considering my general condition and other diseases, what are my blood pressure goals?
- What are my goals in terms of exercise, dietary restrictions, and weight control?
- Are there lifestyle modifications I need to make?
- How will I recognize I am having a heart attack?
- How will I recognize I am having a stroke?
- What should I do if I have any of those symptoms?
- Are there immediate actions I should take before arriving to the emergency department or calling 911?

THINGS YOU CAN DO TO IMPROVE TREATMENT OUTCOMES

- Have a blood pressure monitoring device at home. Measure your blood pressure daily or at least twice a week and keep the records. Try to follow the same pattern when measuring your blood pressure so that your repeated measurements are reliable, for example: similar time of the day, not immediately after activity, after at least 5 minutes of sitting, and on the same arm.
- It is very helpful if you record your systolic and diastolic blood pressure measurements in a table—for example, on a computer spreadsheet. This will allow you to determine objectively whether you are reaching your blood pressure goals. Presenting a spreadsheet printout as a table or a graph to your physician at each follow-up visit will substantially help your

doctor monitor your progress. Remember—the physicians usually only rely on single blood pressure measurements performed in their office and miss all the valuable information in-between. Being proactive and involved with monitoring your treatment goals is going to make your goals more achievable (and your physician happy). There are also various health apps available for smartphone or tablet devices that can help you enter your daily or weekly measured responses and monitor progress.

- Exercise is very important. You don't have to run marathons if you are not in the appropriate condition, but mild to moderate activity for 150 minutes or more per week (as mentioned in Chapter 9) is highly advisable.

- Limit salt intake. High amounts of table salt in the diet can increase your blood pressure.

- Adhere to your medications. Don't miss doses even if you don't have any symptoms and the daily or weekly blood pressure measurements were in the normal range.

- Be cautious with the use of medications for treating nasal congestion or cold—primarily those based on *pseudoephedrine* or similar compounds. They may increase your blood pressure. If you are not sure whether they do, monitor your blood pressure.

- Always keep an updated list of your medications (and their doses) with you. When getting a new prescription from a doctor or acquiring any prescription or nonprescription drug from your pharmacist, always ask if the new medicine interacts with any of your current drugs or can affect your blood pressure. Avoid grapefruit juice if you are taking dihydropyridine calcium channel blockers (e.g., *felodipine*).

VALUABLE RESOURCES FOR ADDITIONAL EDUCATION ON HIGH BLOOD PRESSURE

National Institutes of Health: http://www.nhlbi.nih.gov/health/
health-topics/topics/hbp

Centers for Disease Control and Prevention https://www.cdc.gov/
bloodpressure/

[12]

FIGHTING THE BATTLE
AGAINST LIPIDS
AND CHOLESTEROL

Lipid comes from Greek to describe *fat*. In the context of this chapter, I will refer to *lipids* as naturally occurring fatty molecules such as *cholesterol* and *triglycerides,* which at high concentrations can damage blood vessels and become a risk factor for diseases of the heart and the brain. The condition in which the balance of the blood lipids is disrupted is called *dyslipidemia,* which generally refers to an increase in "bad" cholesterol and in triglycerides and to a decrease in "good" cholesterol. The "bad" cholesterol typical refers to the blood concentration of total cholesterol and of **low-density lipoprotein** (LDL) cholesterol, while "good" cholesterol refers to blood concentration of **high-density lipoprotein** (HDL) cholesterol.

According to a national survey, approximately 50% of the adults in the United States have some kind of dyslipidemia. Even in adults who do not have evidence of current heart or blood vessel disease, about 30% have dyslipidemia. Most people with dyslipidemia have no symptoms, and this lack of symptoms is a good reason to screen for the disease because otherwise it can go undiagnosed and untreated for many years, when it might be too late to intervene effectively.

The biggest risk associated with dyslipidemia is coronary heart disease, or damage to the coronary arteries—the vessels that provide blood and oxygen to the heart. Occlusion (blocking) of the coronary arteries significantly increases the risk for a heart attack and heart failure. The other major risk associated with dyslipidemia is stroke (which results from the occlusion of arteries that deliver blood and oxygen to the brain), although the association between dyslipidemia and stroke is somewhat weaker than with heart disease.

Heart disease is the number one cause of death in the world, and more than half of the deaths due to heart disease are as a result of coronary heart disease that leads to a heart attack (*myocardial infarction*). Fortunately, mortality from heart attacks has been decreasing in the past few decades, indicating that the healthcare system is taking better care of people when they experience a heart attack. However, the number of events (which is the goal of preventive therapy) has been declining at a slower rate compared with mortality rates, meaning that there is still a lot to be done to prevent the coronary events.

TREATMENT GOALS

The main treatment goals in dyslipidemia are to prevent heart disease, heart attacks, and to some extent, stroke. Unfortunately, there is currently no direct way to determine how well the prescribed treatment is working in an individual—that is, what is exactly the success in reducing the individual chance of experiencing a heart attack. We can only assess how the individual is doing compared with the average population. On average, one of every three men will have a heart attack by the age of 75 years. If a man has been treated for dyslipidemia and did not develop heart attack by the age of 75 years, we could assume that the treatment contributed to his health, but we cannot actually measure the extent of this contribution. As in other previously mentioned preventive approaches, we need to rely on surrogate measures to determine whether we are close to achieving the treatment goals.

Several existing surrogate parameters could help us determine how effective the treatment for dyslipidemia is, although there is no single "most important" measure. Similarly to what we discussed about existing goals of optimal blood pressure to prevent complications of hypertension, there are goals for optimal lipid concentrations to prevent complications of dyslipidemia. Currently, the commonly used measures indicating the risk for cardiovascular events associated with dyslipidemia are the blood concentrations (levels) of the following lipids:

- Total cholesterol
- LDL cholesterol
- HDL cholesterol
- Triglycerides

Table 12.1 presents the currently acceptable goals of these lipids in blood, but note that the targets may change depending on your other additional conditions or as new research becomes available.

TREATMENT APPROACH

The approach in general and the treatment goals are somewhat different between people in whom we target *primary prevention* (preventing the **first episode** of heart attack, or stroke, in people with certain risk factors) and those in whom the target is *secondary prevention* (preventing an **additional** episode in someone who already suffered a heart attack or stroke).

TABLE 12.1 GOALS OF LIPID TESTS IN THE TREATMENT
OF DYSLIPIDEMIA

Lipid	Optimal/Near-Optimal Serum* Levels	Levels Clearly Suggesting Increased Risk for Heart Disease	Desired Target Concentrations for Patients at Risk
Total cholesterol	<200 mg/dL	≥240 mg/dL	<200 mg/dL
LDL cholesterol	<100–130 mg/dL[†]	≥160 mg/dL	<70–130 mg/dL[†]
HDL cholesterol	>60 mg/dL	<40 (men) <50 (women)	As high as possible, but >40 mg/dL
Triglycerides	<150 mg/dL	>200 mg/dL	<150–200 mg/dL[†]

*Lipid levels are not measured in the whole blood but rather are measured in **serum** (a part of the blood from which the red blood cells and clotting proteins have been removed).

[†]The target levels depend on additional risk factors such as obesity, smoking, family history, kidney disease, heart disease, and hypertension.

HDL = high-density lipoprotein; LDL = low-density lipoprotein.

There is ample evidence to suggest that high cholesterol levels are associated with increased risk for heart attack, heart disease, and stroke. Beyond the demonstrated association, there also exists a substantial body of research that demonstrates that balancing the blood lipids in patients with risk factors (but who did not have previous events) reduces morbidity and mortality from heart attack and stroke by roughly 10 to 15%. These data mainly come from studies with drugs called *statins*, which I will discuss in detail later in this chapter. The scientific evidence supporting lipid-lowering treatment in patients with established heart disease or after a cardiac event (i.e., secondary prevention) is even stronger than the primary prevention data. In this case, regardless of the actual lipid levels in the blood, therapy with statins is recommended to prevent additional events.

Based on data from more than 170,000 patients, it is evident that for high-risk patients, each 40-mg/dL reduction in LDL cholesterol level is associated with approximately 22% reduction in morbidity and mortality. The optimal duration of treatment for dyslipidemia is not clear, however. The majority of studies have demonstrated positive effects over one- to 10-year treatment periods, with relatively few studies addressing the outcomes beyond the 10-year mark. Nevertheless, in many patients with coronary heart disease or after a heart attack, the physicians will prescribe statins "for life." As long as there is no evidence to the contrary that the long-term treatment is ineffective, it might be reasonable to continue the treatment.

With that said, the potential benefit must be weighed against the risk in each and every individual. If you don't have any side effects from the treatment, and it keeps lipid levels balanced, it is probably reasonable to continue for many years. However, if you have been taking the drug for 20 years, and you are now 87 years old, and the drug causes substantial side effects like headaches and muscle pain, it would be a good idea to discuss the added benefit of that treatment with your doctor. If, for example, the potential benefit is 5% reduction in the risk for heart attack over the next 10 years, in some cases the benefit may not be worth the "cost" of added side effects that impair your quality of life. To be clear—I am not stating this as a recommendation to discontinue statins after 20 years; I am rather raising the point that *pharmacological treatment is not a lifelong contract*. On the contrary, the risks and potential short-term and long-term benefits need to be reassessed as your conditions change or as new research evidence becomes available.

SPECIFIC DRUGS

For achieving the desired lipid levels, several treatment options exist. Before beginning drug treatment, however, it is important to know that some individuals are able to improve lipid balance, and even normalize dyslipidemia, with exercise and diet only. If your body mass index (BMI) is higher than 25, it would be highly advisable to begin an exercise program (or improve the existing one) to achieve normal or near normal weight. Consultation with a dietitian can certainly help to reduce the amount of saturated fats, balance your diet, and achieve optimal weight. And again, as with hypertension, these steps are critical before initiating drug treatment. If exercise, diet, and weight loss are not sufficiently effective, it is then advisable to begin drug therapy for primary prevention. In some circumstances, for example, in genetic (familial) *hypercholesterolemia*, lipid levels may be out of balance even if optimal weight goals are achieved. It is important to note that for secondary prevention, for example, after a heart attack, drug treatment is usually prescribed right away, regardless of weight and the actual serum lipid levels.

Reduction of High Cholesterol Levels

Statins
The most widely used and effective drugs for reducing cholesterol levels are called *HMG-CoA reductase inhibitors*, otherwise known as *statins*. Statins decrease blood cholesterol by inhibiting it's synthesis in the liver. The enzyme HMG-CoA reductase plays a critical role in formation of cholesterol, and by its inhibition, *statins* interfere with

the production of high amounts of cholesterol. Data from a large amount of high-quality studies exist to support the use of statins for the treatment of various types of dyslipidemia.

Several drugs in this family exist, like *simvastatin* (Zocor), *pravastatin* (Pravachol), *atorvastatin* (Lipitor), and *rosuvastatin* (Crestor), to name a few. As you can appreciate, all their generic names end with *statin*. Most statins are taken once a day, and their dose ranges are not very wide: most patients will require "standard" dosing of approximately 20 or 40 mg *simvastatin*, or 10 or 20 mg *atorvastatin*, once a day.

Statins are generally safe drugs if prescribed and taken appropriately; however, there are certain side effects associated with statins that are important to describe. The most common side effect of statins is headache, which occurs in about 5 to 7% of people taking these drugs. It is not necessarily caused by all statins to the same extent. If headaches appear under the treatment of one statin drug, it may be reasonable to switch to a different statin. The headaches are not dangerous but can be unpleasant.

Another important issue to remember is liver enzyme elevation. Changes in liver enzymes, indicating potential liver damage, occur in about 1% of people treated with statins. It is recommended that your doctor performs periodic blood tests to ensure your liver function remains stable. In most cases these changes are not dangerous if diagnosed on time.

Statins may cause muscle pain (myopathy), which may occur in one of every 500 to 1000 patients treated with these medications. In rare cases, this muscle pain can progress to more serious muscle damage, a condition called *rhabdomyolysis*, in which the drug must be immediately discontinued. In rhabdomyolysis, muscle breakdown occurs, and a large amount of protein (which the muscles consist of) is released to the bloodstream, which can damage the kidneys. This is an uncommon complication, occurring in probably less than one of

10,000 people treated with statins. There is a blood test (called creatinine phosphokinase, or CPK) that your doctor may order to test whether there is an indication of muscle damage. Not all statins necessarily cause muscle pain to the same extent, but it is quite clear that the severe cases occur in people who receive high doses of statins and who concomitantly take drugs that increases the statin plasma levels, as described later.

Most statins are metabolized by the cytochrome P-450 (CYP) liver enzyme CYP3A4; therefore, strong inhibitors of the enzyme may increase statin toxicity, increasing the risk for *myopathy* and *rhabdomyolysis*. Several drugs that are CYP3A4 inhibitors must be avoided with statin treatment. Examples include the antifungal medication *itraconazole*, the antibiotic *erythromycin*, and several HIV medications such as *nelfinavir* and *ritonavir*. Other CYP3A4 inhibitors may still cause significant interaction and require a reduction of statin dose or temporary discontinuation. Grapefruit juice, by inhibiting the CYP450 enzyme in the gut, can also increase the toxicity of statins. There are also certain genetic differences among individuals that can determine the risk for developing myopathy. Overall, with moderate doses of statins, and without coadministration of interacting drugs, statin therapy is quite safe, but it is important to consider the previous precautions.

Drugs Other than Statins

Colestipol is a drug that is sometimes used in combination with statins to further reduce blood lipid levels; it is not as effective when used as sole therapy for dyslipidemia. *Colestipol* is taken orally and is not absorbed to the systemic circulation. It binds bile acids in the intestine and increases their excretion through feces. To replace these bile acids, the liver must break down cholesterol, which eventually results in reduction of blood cholesterol levels. The side effects are mainly intestinal and include abdominal discomfort and constipation. The long-term use may cause some blood electrolyte misbalance.

Cholestyramine is chemically different from *colestipol* but works by the same mechanism, by binding bile acids in the intestine. Both *colestipol* and *cholestyramine* may interact with various drugs and reduce their absorption. It is a good idea to consult with a healthcare professional to determine the risk for interactions with your other medications, if you are prescribed either of these two drugs. Because these drugs require physical contact within the intestine to interact, sometimes avoiding the other medications 2 hours before and 4 hours after taking cholestyramine or colestipol will help avoid a negative interaction.

Ezetimibe (Ezetrol, Zetia) is a drug that reduces the absorption of cholesterol, but not the absorption of bile acids like *cholestyramine* and *colestipol* do. It reduces cholesterol levels in blood either alone or in a combination with statins, although the data in support of the effectiveness of *ezetimibe* in preventing heart disease and heart attacks are less convincing than with statins. When used together with statins, *ezetimibe* may increase the risk for liver enzyme elevation and muscle damage. Among the common side effects are diarrhea and abdominal pain. *Ezetimibe* needs to be separated from *cholestyramine* and *colestipol* (2 hours before and 4 hours after their doses). There are ongoing studies to determine the long-term safety of this drug, particularly in combination with statins.

Alirocumab (Praluent) belongs to a new class of drugs called PCSK9 inhibitors. It is given by injection to reduce cholesterol levels and can be an adjunct or alternative for patients in whom statins do not achieve treatment goals or patients who cannot tolerate statins. It's a new medication at this point, and some of the long-term efficacy and safety parameters are not well known.

Lomitapide (Juxtapid) is another recently approved drug, indicated for a relatively small group of patients who have what is called *homozygous familial hypercholesterolemia*—a genetic predisposition to high blood cholesterol levels. The exact role of this drug in the broader population of patients with dyslipidemia is still unclear, but initial data suggest that the drug may have undesirable effects on liver function and has a high potential for drug–drug interactions, including with statins.

To summarize this section, *statins* are the medications with most data by far on long-term safety and effectiveness for treating dyslipidemia. *Cholestyramine* and *colestipol* can be added to the treatment regimen if required, and the newer medications are to be considered on an individual basis, considering the potential risks and benefits of each.

Reduction of High Triglyceride Levels

Although cholesterol is considered one of the main culprits in cardiac disease, triglycerides, the other large component of blood lipids, also have an important role in the development of cardiovascular disorders. Triglycerides are also fatty molecules but have a chemical structure very different from cholesterol, and their synthesis in the body is quite different.

Bezafibrate (Bezalip), *fenofibrate* (Tricor), and *gemfibrozil* (Lopid) are among the drugs used for the treatment of high blood triglyceride levels. These (*fibrate*) drugs reduce triglyceride levels by stimulating lipid breakdown by the liver. In addition to triglyceride reduction, *fibrates* may also reduce LDL cholesterol levels and increase HDL cholesterol levels, although the mechanism for this activity is not clear. Despite being less effective in reducing LDL cholesterol compared with statins, *fibrates* are usually more effective in reducing triglycerides. People with kidney and liver dysfunction may need lower doses or avoid treatment with fibrates, based on the severity of their condition. Among the three, *bezafibrate* is somewhat more effective and has a more favorable side-effect profile.

Bezafibrate is taken orally, usually as a 400-mg sustained-release dose once daily (but can also be prescribed as 200 mg immediate-release tablets). Some skin reactions such as rash or hives may occur with bezafibrate treatment. Most common side effects are intestinal, which may include nausea and abdominal pain. Similarly to other dyslipidemia drugs, bezafibrate may cause an elevation of liver enzymes and increase the risk for myopathy. The risks appear to be small but increases when bezafibrate is combined with statins.

Fenofibrate is taken in a 120- to 160-mg dose, once a day with food. It may negatively affect HDL cholesterol levels, may reduce red and white blood cell counts, and can increase the risk for liver enzyme elevation and myopathy.

Gemfibrozil is administered orally in two daily doses of 600 mg taken 30 minutes before meals. Similarly to *fenofibrate*, it increases the risk for hematologic abnormalities. Red and white blood cell counts may be affected, and periodic monitoring is recommended for timely diagnosis of these abnormalities. Increases in liver enzymes and myopathy are also reported with gemfibrozil, especially when combined with statins.

DRUG-RELATED SPECIAL ISSUES

Proper adherence to *statin* therapy appears to reduce the risk for mortality from heart disease by approximately 30% compared with patients who do not adhere to treatment. Because dyslipidemia is not symptomatic, it is important to make the drug intake a part of your routine so that you don't miss medication doses. The most significant part of cholesterol production by the liver occurs when we are fasting, which means it peaks at night for most people. Therefore, for short-acting statins such as *simvastatin* and *fluvastatin*, the preferred time to take the medicine is before going to sleep so that it is most effective at night. However, statins such as *atorvastatin* and *rosuvastatin* have long half-lives and therefore can be taken anytime during the day.

SPECIAL POPULATIONS

High levels of triglycerides during pregnancy may be associated with some negative pregnancy outcomes, although this might not be true for cholesterol levels. On the other hand, very few clinical studies have assessed the effectiveness and the safety of dyslipidemia drugs in pregnancy. Currently, no drug treatment is recommended in pregnancy. Lifestyle modifications and diet, with a possible addition of omega-3 fatty acids to decrease triglyceride levels, are considered beneficial.

Studies have shown birth defects in offspring of laboratory animals treated with statins during pregnancy. In addition, there have been several case reports of birth defects that might have been associated with maternal statin treatment. With large-scale studies lacking, it is difficult to determine the true risk of statin use in pregnancy. Therefore, the general approach today is to avoid statins during pregnancy. Until new evidence emerges, it is probably the safer approach.

Cholestyramine and *colestipol* are not absorbed and are not expected to directly affect the developing baby (nor are they expected to be problematic during breastfeeding). The potential concern is their indirect effects on the absorption of various lipids and nutrients. No formal safety studies in pregnancy have been performed, and these drugs may be considered if dyslipidemia treatment is important and the expected benefit outweighs the potential risks. There are very few data on the use of fibrates during pregnancy, and they are currently not recommended.

IMPORTANT QUESTIONS TO ASK YOUR DOCTOR

- What are my cholesterol and triglyceride goals?
- What lifestyle changes should I make to help achieve my treatment goals?
- Is there a specific diet recommended for me based on my lipid profile?
- What are the warning sign of risks associated with my current drugs for treating dyslipidemia?
- If I take statins—how can I identify potential myopathy, and what should I do if muscle pain appears?
- Am I taking any drugs that can increase the toxicity of statins (or other drugs I am prescribed for dyslipidemia)?

THINGS YOU CAN DO TO IMPROVE TREATMENT OUTCOMES

- Be sure you are educated about the target levels of your blood lipids.
- Avoid drinking grapefruit juice if you are treated with a statin.
- Before receiving additional drugs—always ask for potential interaction with your dyslipidemia medications.
- If you are overweight—understand that your weight is a significant risk factor for heart disease and complications. Maintaining an exercise and diet program is extremely important for the success of your treatment.
- Be attentive to muscle pain during statin treatment as a potential sign of myopathy. This is not typically pain in a single joint or a small area, but rather is diffuse pain in large muscles

such as the thighs, back, and flanks. If you are uncertain—
stop the treatment and contact your doctor.

VALUABLE RESOURCES FOR ADDITIONAL EDUCATION ON HIGH CHOLESTEROL

The American Heart Association: http://www.heart.org/HEARTORG/
Conditions/Cholesterol/Cholesterol_UCM_001089_SubHome
Page.jsp

Centers for Disease Control and Prevention: https://www.cdc.gov/
cholesterol/

[13]

BLOOD THINNERS

The Balancing Act between Bleeding and Clotting

Meet *hemostasis,* a series of processes with the goal of maintaining blood in its fluid state, inside the blood vessels (not to be confused with *homeostasis*). Hemostasis is of critical importance because it is essentially the ability to form blood clots and prevent excessive blood loss in case of an injury to a blood vessel. In addition, it is the ability to take apart unnecessary blood clots to allow continuous blood flow, which is vital for maintaining body balance (**homeo***stasis*), by proper delivery of oxygen and key molecules to tissues, transporting waste from organs, and regulating body temperature.

Because of the complexity of the clotting system, the introduction for this chapter is going to be somewhat more extensive than for other chapters but is essential for understanding how various blood thinners exert their activity and what conditions they aim to treat or prevent.

BLOOD AND CLOTTING

Let's briefly discuss what blood consists of and how various drugs can affect its clotting. As illustrated in Figure 13.1, blood is composed of (1) plasma, (2) red blood cells, (3) white blood cells, and (4) platelets (which technically are not cells, but cell fragments). Plasma is the liquid without cells, that is, the blood from which cells and platelets have been removed. Plasma contains a variety of molecules and proteins and is rich in **coagulation factors** (or clotting factors), a group of molecules that are critical for blood clotting.

Our body has two main mechanisms for limiting blood loss following an injury to blood vessels, and these two mechanisms work in concert, simultaneously:

1. Activation of platelets, which causes them to clump together, forming a plug that blocks the injury site to minimize blood loss.

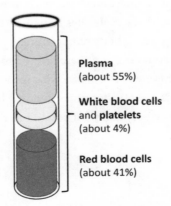

Plasma
(about 55%)

White blood cells
and **platelets**
(about 4%)

Red blood cells
(about 41%)

Figure 13.1. Composition of the whole blood. Plasma contains the clotting factors. Plasma with the clotting factors removed is called *serum*.

2. Activation of various *coagulation factors* in plasma to eventually form *fibrin*. Fibrin is a key protein in clotting; when multiple fibrin units bind to each other, they form a clotting mesh. This fibrin mesh, together with clumped platelets, forms the eventual clot (or plug) over the injured blood vessel.

Most blood-thinning drugs target one of the above two mechanisms: they either have **antiplatelet** activity (inhibit platelet clumping, or platelet *aggregation*), or **anticoagulant** activity (interfere with one or more of the *coagulation factors* to prevent the formation of *fibrin*).

CONDITIONS OF EXCESSIVE BLOOD CLOTTING

In several conditions, excessive platelet clumping (aggregation) and blood clotting lead to morbidity and sometimes death. In a somewhat simplistic manner, I will discuss the two major types of complications associated with formation of a clot (*thrombus*) within a blood vessel.

The *first type* is associated with *atherosclerosis*, a fatty streak that runs along the blood vessels. Smoking, high blood cholesterol levels, high blood pressure, and obesity are all associated with increased risk for atherosclerosis. Atherosclerosis is particularly dangerous when the blood vessels involved are the ones that supply blood to critically important organs such as the heart and the brain. These fatty streaks inside the blood vessels narrow down the diameter available for blood flow but also attract various lipids and debris to "stick" to it and further narrow the space through which the blood can flow.

Damage to the blood vessel or a rupture of that *atherosclerotic* streak can trigger platelet aggregation and clotting mechanisms, which, in turn, can completely block the blood supply to a section of an organ, creating an *infarct,* a localized area of dead tissue. If large enough, these infarcts in heart or brain tissues are fatal. In fact, the process I just described is one of the most common mechanisms by which a **heart attack** (*myocardial* infarction, or the block of blood supply to the heart muscle) or a **stroke** (*cerebral* infarction, or the block of blood supply to the brain tissue) occurs.

The *second type* of complication is associated with *thromboembolism,* a process that creates a blood clot (*thrombus*) in a vessel, followed by the detachment of a piece of that thrombus, which travels in the direction of blood flow and then blocks the passage of the blood in a vessel in a different part of the body. This obstruction in blood flow is called an *embolus* (plural—*emboli*). Certain conditions increase the risk for forming such a clot. *Atrial fibrillation,* which is a certain type of heart rhythm abnormality, is one of the most common causes. *Atrial fibrillation* increases the risk for clot-forming in the heart or in one of the blood vessels of the heart. A piece of that clot can detach from its origin (as described earlier), travel through the bloodstream to the brain, and cause serious damage by creating *emboli* in the brain. The complication of such a process will be a **stroke,** and clinically, it would be quite similar to the *atherosclerotic* stroke described in the previous paragraph because the net result in both cases is the obstruction of blood supply to a portion of the brain.

Similarly to how clots are formed in the case of atrial fibrillation, a variety of conditions can increase the risk for what is called *venous thromboembolism,* where the clots are formed in the veins, especially of the legs. Among factors that increase the risk for thromboembolism are surgeries (especially orthopedic surgeries of lower limbs), pregnancy, use of oral contraceptives (especially in smoking women older than 35 years), cancer, obesity, and trauma, to name a few. After a thrombus is formed in a vein, a similar process of detachment and embolization can create a life-threatening condition if the thrombus clogs a blood vessel supplying blood to organs such as the lungs, the brain, the heart, or the kidneys. Foreign objects that come in contact with blood, such as artificial heart valves, can further increase the risk for such embolic events.

Now that we have discussed the background on hemostasis and the complications associated with excessive blood clotting, we can move to the main objective of this chapter, which is to discuss the pharmacological therapy for preventing *atherosclerotic* and *thromboembolic* events. These treatments are aimed at preventing heart attacks, strokes, emboli in the lungs (called *pulmonary emboli*), and other serious complications of excessive blood clotting.

Heart attacks (acute *myocardial infarction*, abbreviated as **MI**) are still among the leading causes of death: every year about 735,000 Americans have a heart attack (more than one heart attack every minute). Although the mortality rates from a heart attack seem to be declining since 2010 or so, about 250,000 to 300,000 people a year still die from a heart attack in the United States alone. There are probably a few reasons for the mortality decline. First, the rate of smoking has decreased, and the positive effects of smoking bans have started to emerge. Second, effective preventive therapies, combined with in-hospital fast-paced interventions, are successfully (but slowly) driving the mortality rates down.

Stroke is another deadly condition relevant to this chapter. Almost 800,000 people a year in the United States have a stroke, 130,000 of whom die. That's about one person every 4 minutes. Stroke is the leading cause of long-term serious disability, and costs an estimated $34 billion to the US economy every year. Although there are several types of strokes, the ones associated with obstructed blood flow to the brain, as described earlier, account for about 75% of the cases. The prevention of a stroke among patients with *atrial fibrillation* is one of the main reasons patients receive blood-thinning therapy. Currently, about 3.2 million people in the United States have atrial fibrillation, and its prevalence has been increasing. The recognition and management of atrial fibrillation is important because it increases the risk for stroke by about five-fold.

In addition to heart attacks and strokes, almost 1 million thromboembolic events, such as blood clots in the lungs or in the veins of the legs, occur annually in the United States, with $13 billion to $27 billion associated direct and indirect costs. There are additional conditions for which your doctor may prescribe anticoagulant treatment for you, such as genetic and immune-mediated coagulation disorders, but these will not be discussed separately in this chapter.

TREATMENT GOALS

Since preventing excessive blood clotting has a different utility in each of the previously discussed conditions, the treatment goals will be different in each case. For primary or secondary prevention of a heart attack—the goal would be precisely that—preventing the first (or the next) heart attack. The same parallel can be drawn for preventing thrombotic or embolic events in primary or secondary prevention of stroke.

The goal is **prevention**, as in dyslipidemia and hypertension. You can guess already—measuring the success of anticoagulant treatment is going to be challenging on an individual level, and in some cases we are going to use surrogate measures to help us determine how effective the treatment is.

For *antiplatelet* treatments, such as aspirin, there is no objective measure to tell us how close we are to attaining our preventive goal, or how close we are to the risk for excessive bleeding. For some anticoagulant treatments, there are surrogate measures of clotting and bleeding (tests called activated partial thromboplastin time [aPTT] and international normalized ratio [INR], which I will discuss shortly) that can help guide the treatment. In fact, the treatment goals will be to achieve the therapeutic range of INR recommended for the specific condition.

TREATMENT APPROACH

In primary prevention, when people may not have any symptoms, the healthcare providers and screening programs seek to identify the high-risk individuals in the community and to minimize those risk factors that can be modified, like excessive weight, smoking, high blood pressure, heart disease, high blood cholesterol levels, excessive calorie intake in diet, and sedentary lifestyle. If required, blood-thinning treatment will be prescribed based on the presence of these risk factors. As an individual, understanding these risk factors and seeking medical advice early can help prevent or decrease the risk for serious complications.

The main risk in atherosclerosis is a thrombotic infarct in the heart or the brain; therefore, in high-risk individuals, therapy for inhibiting platelet aggregation, such as treatment with *aspirin*, would typically be appropriate. If you happen to have atrial fibrillation, which increases the risk for embolic stroke, then *anticoagulant* treatment with drugs such as *warfarin* (Coumadin), *factor Xa inhibitors* (e.g., *apixaban* or *rivaroxaban*), or *direct thrombin inhibitors* (e.g., *dabigatran*) may be indicated. See Table 13.1 for a summary of antiplatelet and anticoagulant drugs.

Patients who already had a stroke, a heart attack, or another thromboembolic event are clearly at high risk for a second event, so all of them should receive secondary prevention. The drugs for secondary prevention also belong to either the antiplatelet or anti-coagulant category used for primary prevention, although the treatment might be a bit more "aggressive" (i.e., using higher doses or a combination of drugs). The specific medication, its dose, and the

TABLE 13.1 SUMMARY OF ANTIPLATELET AND ANTICOAGULANT DRUGS

Antiplatelet Drug(s)	Route of Administration and Doses	Type of Monitoring beyond Routine Signs of Bleeding	Drug Interactions	Tips for Administration
Aspirin Aspirin inhibits an enzyme called COX, which is responsible for producing thromboxane, which helps platelets aggregate. Less thromboxane leads to less platelet clumping	Usually 50–325 mg/day in a single oral dose	Usually no special monitoring, besides signs of bleeding	Steroids, NSAIDs, and SSRI drugs for depression may increase the risk for GI bleeding. If you need to take ibuprofen (and possibly other NSAIDs), take it *after* the daily aspirin dose*	Usually with meals, although with enteric-coated formulations (see Chapter 4), this is probably not critical
Thienopyridines—clopidogrel (Plavix), *ticlopidine* (Ticlid), and *prasugrel* (Effient) Thienopyridines require activation in the liver, after which they inhibit a receptor on platelets that is called the PY_{12} receptor (or ADP receptor). This mechanism is different from that of aspirin, but the effect is similar—inhibition of platelet aggregation	*Clopidogrel* (most commonly used) and *prasugrel* are taken orally once a day; *ticlopidine* twice a day	Usually no special monitoring, besides signs of bleeding *Ticlopidine* may cause blood cell abnormalities—frequent blood counts should be performed. *Clopidogrel* rarely causes serious blood cell abnormalities	*Omeprazole,** and possibly other inhibitors of CYP2C19 (e.g., *fluconazole* [Diflucan], *fluoxetine* [Prozac]), can decrease effectiveness of *clopidogrel*	Might be appropriate to perform genetic testing* of CYP enzyme function before initiating treatment with *clopidogrel*

Dipyridamole				
The antiplatelet effect of *dipyridamole* is different from that of aspirin and of thienopyridines. It inhibits an enzyme called *phosphodiesterase* and inhibits platelet aggregation by a different mechanism. It also enhances the effect of aspirin	Either administered in a combined capsule with *aspirin* (Aggrenox) to be taken twice a day, or *dipyridamole* alone (Persantine) 3–4 times a day for the prevention of thromboembolism	Usually requires no monitoring. Important side effects: chest pain, rash	Interacts with other drugs that can enhance bleeding—other anticoagulants, aspirin, NSAIDs, SSRI/SNRI antidepressants	Absorption may differ among different formulations. Preferably take on empty stomach. If the drug causes upset stomach, then take with food
Warfarin (Coumadin) and derivatives (*acenocoumarol*) Vitamin K is necessary for proper functioning of several coagulation factors. These drugs essentially act as vitamin K antagonists and interfere with production of functional coagulation factors	Dose based on INR.* Usually dose in the range of 2–10 mg/day, taken once a day Some people may require different doses on different weekdays to achieve optimal INR	INR monitoring. Usually recommended INR is ~2.5 (generally in the range between 2 and 3)	*Warfarin* interacts with ***many*** drugs. It is metabolized by CYP enzymes in the liver, particularly by CYP2C9. Various CYP inhibitors or inducers may increase or decrease its effect, respectively Dietary supplements: *ginkgo* can increase anticoagulant effect; *St. John's wort* can decrease effect	Avoid activities that may result in cuts or bruising. Use soft toothbrush. Don't make drastic changes in the consumption of green vegetables such as broccoli, asparagus, spinach (all rich in vitamin K). Consuming large quantities of **pomegranate** juice or **cranberry** juice may increase the risk for bleeding with warfarin

(*continued*)

TABLE 13.1 CONTINUED

Antiplatelet Drug(s)	Route of Administration and Doses	Type of Monitoring beyond Routine Signs of Bleeding	Drug Interactions	Tips for Administration
Factor Xa inhibitors—apixaban (Eliquis), *rivaroxaban* (Xarelto), *edoxaban* (Savaysa) These drugs specifically inhibit factor Xa, one of the key coagulation factors in the formation of thrombin	*Apixaban*: Orally, twice a day *Rivaroxaban*: Orally, once or twice a day, depending on indication *Edoxaban*: Orally, once a day Main side effects are associated with excessive bleeding. Additional effects include rash and itching.	Usually no need for monitoring. *Edoxaban* loses some of its effects when kidney function is completely normal (the drug is cleared quickly from bloodstream)	Grapefruit juice may increase bleeding with *apixaban*. In general, a variety of interactions with CYP enzyme inducers and inhibitors. Extra caution required. *Rivaroxaban*: Taking CYP 3A4 inhibitors such as *ketoconazole* and *ritonavir* can increase toxicity	These drugs may be prescribed after knee or hip replacement surgeries to prevent thrombosis Missed dose should be taken as soon as possible
Direct thrombin inhibitors— *dabigatran* (Pradaxa), *desirudin* (Iprivask) These drugs inhibit thrombin (factor IIa), another key factor in the coagulation process	*Dabigatran*: Orally, twice a day *Desirudin*: Injected under the skin, twice a day, for thrombosis prevention after surgery	High risk for bleeding. Monitoring not mandatory but can be useful. aPTT is more accurate than INR monitoring in the case of *dabigatran*	*Dabigatran*: Antifungal *ketoconazole* and certain HIV medications can increase toxicity of *dabigatran*. Combination with NSAIDs and certain antidepressants increase the risk for bleeding	Both *dabigatran* and *desirudin* should be used with caution or avoided in kidney impairment (depending on the degree of kidney damage)

Low-molecular-weight heparin (LMWH)—*enoxaparin* (Lovenox, Clexane), *dalteparin* (Fragmin). *Fondaparinux* (Arixtra) is a *factor Xa inhibitor* but is administered similarly to LMWH	*Enoxaparin:* Injected under the skin, once or twice a day *Dalteparin:* Various dosing regimens exist—generally around 2500–10,000 units injected under the skin once a day *Fondaparinux:* Injected under the skin, once a day	With all three drugs, blood counts should be periodically performed because they can negatively affect blood cell and platelet counts. Anti–factor Xa levels may be monitored for efficacy	Drug–drug interactions are primarily with other anticoagulants. These drugs are excreted mostly by kidney; practically no drug interactions based on liver metabolism	*Dalteparin* injection may cause local pain and irritation Thrombocytopenia (reduction of number of platelets in the blood) may occur with any of the three drugs. This requires monitoring *Fondaparinux* and *enoxaparin* are not to be administered if platelet count falls below 100,000. People who weigh less than 50 kg (110 lb) and people with kidney impairment are at excess risk for bleeding

*Details are available in the text.

aPTT = activated partial thromboplastin time; GI = gastrointestinal; INR = international normalized ratio; NSAID = nonsteroidal anti-inflammatory drug; SNRI = serotonin–norepinephrine reuptake inhibitor; SSRI = selective serotonin reuptake inhibitor.

duration of treatment are chosen on an individual basis, considering the current evidence on the specific type of thromboembolic event, the patient's other conditions, and the overall risk for a recurrent event. After a heart attack, your doctor may prescribe, for example, *clopidogrel* for 6 months and then lifelong therapy with low-dose *aspirin*. Alternatively, your doctor may initiate treatment with *warfarin* (Coumadin) indefinitely, if the immediate risk is high. If you have clots in your deep veins (typically in the legs or pelvis) or have atrial fibrillation, you may be prescribed *warfarin* or other groups of medications such as *low-molecular-weight heparin* (LMWH; e.g., *enoxaparin* or *dalteparin*), a *factor Xa inhibitor*, or a *direct thrombin inhibitor*. The guidelines for effective primary and secondary prevention change from time to time as new evidence and new drugs become available.

Keep in mind that some strokes are caused by excessive bleeding (*hemorrhagic* stroke) rather than excessive clotting. In these cases, blood-thinning therapy for secondary prevention will not be warranted. Based on the conditions that led to the stroke, your doctor will decide which approach for secondary prevention is appropriate. If you experienced a stroke, it would be important to ask your doctor which of the two types of stroke you had so that you better understand the approach for preventing the next stroke.

It is important to remember that blood-thinning is a double-edged sword; the further you move from clotting, the closer you get to bleeding. It ALWAYS requires a delicate balance, preferably under the guidance of an experienced physician. The key to success is in optimizing the treatment to reach the "Goldilocks principle" of sufficient prevention of clotting, without causing excessive bleeding.

The National Action Plan for Adverse Drug Event Prevention (ADE Action Plan) has identified anticoagulants among the three most significant areas of patient safety concern with medications (together with agents for treating diabetes and opioids for treating pain).

Because of the delicate balance between clotting and bleeding, safe and effective anticoagulation requires very efficient teamwork between the patient and the healthcare providers. Properly educating yourself on how anticoagulants work and how they cause toxicity is an important topic for achieving optimal treatment outcomes.

SPECIFIC DRUGS

There are multiple classes of drugs to prevent clotting and also drugs to help dissolve clots that are in formation. A few of these are administered by injection in hospitalized patients, for example, after a heart attack or stroke, or in relation to a surgery or critical illness. Since their administration is typically initiated and performed by the medical team, with no active participation of the patient, I will not be discussing these anticoagulant and antithrombotic treatments in this chapter. The focus will rather be on medications that you would get at home.

DRUG-RELATED SPECIAL ISSUES

With any antiplatelet or anticoagulant drug treatment, it is of extreme importance to *monitor for signs of bleeding*. These signs include very easily bruised skin, nosebleeds, bleeding gums when toothbrushing, blood in urine or feces, anemia, and tiredness. Symptoms of ineffective anticoagulation would be those of thrombosis, which is most common in the feet: leg pain, swelling, redness, tenderness to touch, and warmth.

The first drugs to discuss in this section are *aspirin* and other *nonsteroidal anti-inflammatory drugs (NSAIDs)*. Aspirin is an NSAID that works by inhibiting an enzyme called cyclooxygenase (COX) that is responsible for the formation of *thromboxane,* which promotes platelet aggregation, and other molecules that promote inflammation and pain (see Chapter 18 for more detail). At high doses, aspirin can be used to reduce pain and inflammation, but aspirin and other NSAIDs can also inhibit platelet aggregation and can increase the risk for bleeding. The main difference that gives aspirin its advantage in preventing strokes and heart attacks is the fact that is binds permanently (*irreversibly*) to the COX enzyme and basically neutralizes the ability of a platelet to function for a few days. The effect of aspirin on platelets can be achieved by low doses (typically 75 to 325 mg), without the need of administering high analgesic doses (around 2000 mg/day). The effect of aspirin on platelets weans off only when new fresh platelets are produced by the bone marrow. This is in contrast to NSAIDs, which inhibit COX only temporarily, for a few hours. When you take an NSAID, such as ibuprofen, within a couple of hours *before* taking aspirin, the ibuprofen is now bound temporarily to the platelets, and aspirin cannot act on the enzyme because COX is "busy" binding to the ibuprofen. In the opposite scenario, when aspirin is taken first, it "inactivates" the platelets by irreversible binding, and taking ibuprofen an hour or later after aspirin will not diminish the effect of aspirin on platelets.

Bottom line: if you take daily aspirin for platelet inhibition and you need to take another NSAID for relieving pain or inflammation, then (1) consult your doctor about the added risk for stomach or intestinal bleeding with the combination and (2) take your aspirin at least 1 hour *before* (or at least 8 hours *after*) your other NSAID such as *ibuprofen. Acetaminophen* is probably a safer choice, if analgesic (not anti-inflammatory) therapy is indicated in aspirin users because acetaminophen does not inhibit the COX enzyme.

Clopidogrel (Plavix) is a newer antiplatelet agent. In some conditions it is more effective than aspirin or is prescribed to individuals who cannot take aspirin because of allergies or other reasons. To exert its action, *clopidogrel* requires activation by a liver cytochrome enzyme called CYP2C19. Some people genetically produce a modified version of 2C19 enzyme, and in this group of patients, *clopidogrel* is less effective and may not protect them from excessive blood clotting. Your doctor may decide to perform genetic testing before prescribing clopidogrel.

Several observational studies suggested that taking medications like *omeprazole* (Prilosec), which reduces acidity in the stomach, decreases the efficacy of *clopidogrel* by affecting its metabolism through CYP2C19 enzyme inhibition. In 2009, the US Food and Drug Administration (FDA) issued a warning recommending against the combination of *omeprazole* and *clopidogrel*. While new evidence from well-conducted studies suggests that the interaction may not be as significant as it was previously thought to be, in November 2016 the FDA reissued the recommendation against the combination. Because data on the topic may change with newer studies becoming available, the decision will be made on an individual basis. If treatment for stomach acidity is required in a clopidogrel-treated individual, other drugs from this group (e.g., *pantoprazole*) with a lower CYP2C19-inhibitory effect may be a safer option.

Warfarin (Coumadin) is one of the most common anticoagulant drugs, especially effective in preventing stroke and other thromboembolic events in atrial fibrillation and thrombosis in deep veins. More than 30 million *warfarin* prescriptions are written annually in the United States. In atrial fibrillation, *warfarin* treatment reduces the chance of stroke by 50 to 80%. On the other hand, the frequency of bleeding is 15 to 20% greater per year (one of every five to seven treated patients), and the frequency of life-threatening or fatal bleeding is increased by 1 to 3% per year (one of every 30 to 100 patients).

One of the most important measures to indicate the extent of anticoagulation with *warfarin* is a blood test for INR, which indicates the extent of blood clotting. The normal INR is around 1. With *warfarin* therapy, the target range in most cases would be between 2 and 3 INR and in some cases up to 3.5 INR. Higher INR values usually increase the risk for bleeding. In cases in which the INR is too high, or in *warfarin* overdose cases, the physician may prescribe *vitamin K* (by mouth or by injection) to reduce the risk for bleeding.

Several *new oral anticoagulant (NOAC)* drugs have been developed in recent years. These include *dabigatran* (factor IIa inhibitor) and *rivaroxaban, apixaban,* and *edoxaban* (factor Xa inhibitors). Largely, these drugs are alternatives to *warfarin.* While *warfarin,* by interfering with vitamin K activity, affects the function of half a dozen coagulation factors that are dependent on *vitamin K,* NOAC drugs affect more specific proteins in the coagulation process. In studies comparing NOACs with warfarin, the two had similar effects on preventing thromboembolic events such as stroke, with a somewhat lower risk for major bleeding with NOACs. NOAC generally do not require monitoring (e.g., frequent INR tests, as with warfarin), but at this point in time they are substantially more expensive than the generic *warfarin.* The individual choice of the appropriate anticoagulation therapy needs to take into account the various individual risk factors and existing conditions.

LMWHs, such as *enoxaparin* or *dalteparin,* also lead to inhibition of coagulation factors, mainly of factor Xa. In the out-of-hospital setting, these drugs are mainly used for the prevention of thrombosis in deep veins (legs and pelvis)—often in high-risk pregnancies, in people who are bed bound, and in those with certain types of cancers where risk for thrombosis is high. LMWH drugs are administered by a subcutaneous injection (under the skin), typically once or twice a day. The most common injection site is the abdomen; it is recommended to rotate the injection sites to reduce skin irritation. In people with kidney failure, dose adjustments or other forms of heparin may be indicated. LMWH may cause anemia and reduction in the platelet counts.

SPECIAL POPULATIONS

All anticoagulant and antiplatelet medications have a higher risk for causing bleeding in (1) older adults; (2) people undergoing surgical or interventional procedures, such as epidural injections; and (3) people with gastrointestinal conditions, such as stomach ulcers.

Pregnant women with certain conditions may have an increased risk for thromboembolic events. Pregnancy itself causes a five-fold increase in the risk for thrombosis in deep veins. While in most pregnancies there is no need for thrombosis prevention with drugs, this can be required in certain high-risk pregnancies. In these cases, the preferential treatment is usually with *LMWHs*, which do not cross the placenta to affect the fetus. *Warfarin* is known for increasing the risk for birth defects, especially if used during the sixth to 12th weeks of pregnancy. *Warfarin* may be considered against *LMWH* in unique situations, but the optimal approach and regimen should be discussed with your physician.

Patients on chronic selective serotonin reuptake inhibitor (*SSRI*) antidepressant therapy and taking *corticosteroids* or *NSAIDs* are at an increased risk for bleeding, especially stomach bleeds, when receiving additional antiplatelet or anticoagulant therapy. The benefit of these drugs should be weighted carefully against the possible risk for bleeding. Stomach protection (with medications such as *omeprazole* or *pantoprazole*), more frequent monitoring, or alternative treatment strategies should be discussed with the treating physician.

IMPORTANT QUESTIONS TO ASK YOUR DOCTOR

- What are my treatment goals?
- How long do I need to receive this treatment?
- What drugs, foods, and drinks should I avoid with my current treatment?
- How can I identify signs of bleeding or too much coagulation (thrombosis)?
- What should I do if I notice signs of bleeding or thrombosis?

THINGS YOU CAN DO TO IMPROVE TREATMENT OUTCOMES

- Don't stop antiplatelet or anticoagulant therapy without consulting your doctor. Sudden discontinuation can increase the risk for blood clots, which can be life-threatening.
- If you need to get periodic monitoring, such as INR or blood count, make sure you do not skip the tests, and ask your doctor about test results and what they mean for you and your treatment plan.
- Notify your medical team that you are on blood-thinning medications every time you are to undergo a surgical or medical procedure, including epidural injections or dental work, because you are at increased risk for bleeding.
- Make the maximum effort not to skip or double your doses. Sometimes, especially with *warfarin* therapy, you might be prescribed to take different doses on different days to achieve a certain weekly dose, for example, one 5 mg pill every day, but an extra half pill on Mondays and Thursdays.

VALUABLE RESOURCES FOR ADDITIONAL EDUCATION ON ANTICOAGULATION

Centers for Disease Control and Prevention: http://www.cdc.gov/
stroke/facts.htm and http://www.cdc.gov/ncbddd/dvt/facts.
html

National Blood Clot Alliance: https://www.stoptheclot.org/learn_
more/about-clots.htm

[14]

NOT SO SWEET

Managing Diabetes

Diabetes comes from Greek, meaning "siphon" or "excessive discharge of urine." Later on, the word *mellitus* (*sweet* in Latin) was added to the formal medical term, *diabetes mellitus* (DM) primarily because of the high concentration of sugar in the urine of diabetic patients. There are two major types of DM: type 1 and type 2. Type 1 (previously called juvenile diabetes mellitus) is characterized by damage to the pancreas by our own immune cells, which results in the inability of the pancreas to produce insulin, the hormone that controls sugar (glucose) levels in the blood. Type 2 diabetes (previously called adult-onset diabetes) is characterized by "resistance to insulin," which means that normal release of insulin is unable to control blood sugar levels by moving it from the blood to various tissues that need it. As a consequence of this resistance to insulin, the pancreas is required to produce more insulin to control blood sugar. Unfortunately, this is typically a progressive process in type 2 diabetes, and the resistance worsens over time, requiring more and more insulin production, to the point that the pancreas reaches a limit and is unable to produce enough insulin to keep the blood sugar levels within normal range.

I will focus on type 2 diabetes here and discuss both insulin and noninsulin treatments. Since type 1 diabetes is characterized by lack of insulin production, it is treated almost exclusively by insulin; therefore, the principles of insulin therapy I will discuss for type 2 DM generally apply to type 1 DM as well. *Gestational diabetes* is an additional type of diabetes that appears during pregnancy, but this is outside the scope of the current chapter.

Diabetes affects about 30 million people in the United States alone, which is more than 9% of the population. For those older than 65 years, the prevalence of diabetes is estimated to be 27%, which is predominantly type 2 DM. The prevalence of diabetes is affected by weight: in people with normal weight, the prevalence of diabetes is about 2 to 3%, but in individuals whose weight is 40% over their ideal weight, this prevalence increases to about 10%. DM is characterized by increased sugar (glucose) in the blood and is caused by a mix of several factors, including genetic and environmental ones.

Insulin is a hormone synthesized and secreted by the pancreas, an organ that is located under the stomach. The role of insulin is to control growth and development, primarily by controlling the entry of glucose from the bloodstream into the cells in various tissues. If glucose from the bloodstream does not enter effectively into the cells, it will accumulate in the blood, and the tissues will not get enough glucose. Glucose is an important source of energy for many tissues and almost an exclusive source of energy for the brain.

In healthy people, the pancreas constantly releases a certain amount of insulin (called *basal rate*), and when glucose levels in the blood are high, for example, after a meal, the pancreas releases more insulin to the blood in order to help move glucose from the blood to other tissues, such as the liver, the brain, and the muscles. This process has two purposes. One, the tissues need glucose as energy source, and two, excessive levels of glucose in blood can damage the blood vessels. In diabetes, not only is the production of insulin in the pancreas impaired, but tissues also become resistant to insulin. This means that, without an intervention, glucose concentration in the blood is going to be high because the mechanism that helps get rid of excess sugar in the blood is damaged.

Diabetes is quite a horrid disease. The high circulating levels of glucose in the blood harm many organs, mainly through damaging small and large blood vessels that supply blood to these organs. Diabetes can damage the heart, the eyes, the kidneys, and various nerves in the body, like the nerves innervating the gut, and small nerve fibers responsible for sensation. By damaging both blood vessels and nerves in the genital organs, diabetes is a frequent cause of erectile dysfunction in men. I provide these excessive details to highlight our subsequent discussion on multiple goals that diabetic patients may need to achieve.

TREATMENT GOALS

Owing to incredible scientific progress, achieving normal or near-normal quality of life and life-expectancy in diabetes today is a possibility, which would have been an elusive dream just a few decades ago. With that said, diabetic patients often need to make a substantial effort to prevent blood vessel damage, kidney damage, eye damage, and nerve damage in order to achieve these goals. A tight control of blood glucose levels may help in preventing many of the complications altogether, but monitoring the function of the eyes, kidneys, heart, and nerves is going to be important for determining the success of the therapy.

There are immediate and long-term goals of DM therapy. Among the *immediate (short-term) goals* are the following:

- To prevent extremely high glucose levels that could cause a life-threatening situation. This situation, termed *diabetic ketoacidosis* (DKA), is more frequent in type 1 DM but can also occur in type 2 DM. It is characterized by severe electrolyte imbalance and dehydration and requires immediate hospitalization. The symptoms you may experience if you have DKA include excessive thirst, frequent urination, abdominal pain, nausea, weakness, fruity-scented breath, and confusion. DKA can be life-threatening; overall mortality from DKA is about 1%, but in older adult patients with many other medical conditions, it can be as high as 5% (one death out of 20 hospital admissions for DKA).

- Another short-term goal is to prevent hypoglycemia, a drop in blood glucose levels (typically to lower than 70 mg/dL). Serious hypoglycemia is considered when glucose levels drop under 40 mg/dL, or the hypoglycemic patient requires third-party assistance (family member or medical personnel). Hypoglycemia may cause poor concentration and coordination, dizziness, confusion, and even coma. Hypoglycemia may be triggered by medications (frequently injection of insulin without an appropriate meal), exercise, stress, or other factors.

The *long-term goals* of diabetes treatment are to prevent organ damage, primarily heart and kidney disease but also, as mentioned, damage to the eyes, the nerves, and the digestive tract. Diabetes is also a risk factor for other diseases such as high blood pressure and dyslipidemia, so good glucose control can help prevent these complications as well.

The treatment plan for diabetes needs to focus on achieving good control of blood glucose, while preventing very high and very low glucose levels. Glucose levels in the blood can be determined by a laboratory test or a home glucose test. A special test called hemoglobin A_{1c} (HbA_{1c}) will provide information on the average glucose levels in your blood during 3 months before the test. HbA_{1c}

testing requires a blood draw, which is usually done in a lab or the physician's office. Generally, HbA_{1c} level between 3 and 6 is considered normal, and HbA_{1c} level below 7 is a desired target for most people with diabetes. Consult your doctor on how frequently this test needs to be performed to help you achieve optimal treatment results.

TREATMENT APPROACH

Similarly to treating dyslipidemia (see Chapter 12), the treatment of DM frequently requires a combination of pharmacological and nonpharmacological treatments. In overweight or obese individuals, controlled weight loss can greatly improve glucose control. This should be obtained by building an exercise routine (based on your capability) and maintaining low-carbohydrate diet. These lifestyle modifications can substantially help control your glucose level; nevertheless, drug therapy will often be required.

Several groups of medications exist for treating type 2 diabetes, most administered orally. Some medications work by stimulating the release of insulin from the pancreas, which helps move glucose from the blood to the cells. Others work by suppressing glucose production by the liver and by reducing the resistance (increasing the sensitivity) of tissues to insulin. The mechanisms by which the various medication classes help control glucose levels are summarized in Table 14.1. In people whose glucose levels do not normalize with oral medications, or those who for various reasons do not tolerate oral medications (e.g., because of side effects), it may make sense to start insulin therapy. In some cases insulin will be combined with oral drugs, and in others treatment will be based on insulin only. In type 1 diabetes, the therapy is primarily insulin based, although in certain cases the addition of a drug called *metformin* (see Table 14.1 for

TABLE 14.1 NONINSULIN DRUGS USED TO TREAT DIABETES MELLITUS

Examples of Drugs	Method of Administration	Drug Class	Mechanism	Relation to Food
Glyburide or glibenclamide* (Daonil, Micronase), glipizide (Gluco-Rite)	Oral	Sulfonylureas—second generation	Stimulate insulin secretion from the pancreas	Take immediately before or with a meal to prevent hypoglycemia
Chlorpropamide (Diabinese), tolbutamide (Orinase). (These drugs are not often used now)	Oral	Sulfonylureas—second generation	Stimulate insulin secretion from the pancreas	Take with a meal to prevent hypoglycemia
Metformin (Glucophage, others)	Oral	Biguanides	Inhibit glucose production by the liver, increase the sensitivity of peripheral tissues to insulin	Take with or after food to prevent abdominal pain and bloating
Acarbose (Precose, Prandase)	Oral	Alpha-glucosidase inhibitors	Reduce the amount of carbohydrates (sugar) from the gut to the blood	Only works if taken with meals that include carbohydrates

Drug (brand)	Route	Class	Mechanism	When to take
Sitagliptin (Januvia) Linagliptin (Tradjenta)	Oral	Dipeptidyl peptidase-4 inhibitor	Inhibit the release of glucagon hormone from the pancreas (which increases glucose levels)	With or without food
Rosiglitazone (Avandia)	Oral	Thiazolidinediones	Mechanism not completely understood. Assumed to reduce insulin resistance in fat tissues	With or without food
Exenatide (Byetta), liraglutide (Victoza), dulaglutide (Trulicity), albiglutide (Tanzeum)	Injectable	Incretin mimetics	Mimic the action of glucagon-like peptide 1 (GLP-1). GLP-1 is a molecule released from the gut in response to food intake and acts as a hormone	Within 60 minutes before a meal
Empagliflozin (Jardiance), dapagliflozin (Farxiga), and canagliflozin (Invokana)	Oral	Gliflozins, or sodium glucose co-transporter 2 (SGLT2) inhibitors	Enhances glucose excretion in urine by inhibiting sodium reabsorption from kidneys	With or without food

*Glyburide and glibenclamide are both generic names of the same drug molecule.

details) may be appropriate because it may improve the sensitivity of tissues to insulin.

The major types of insulin are outlined in Table 14.2. Some insulin types act rapidly, within 15 or 30 minutes, but last only a few hours, while others begin their effect more slowly but last longer. In recent years, several types of long-acting insulin have been developed, with the effect lasting for about 24 hours, allowing once-daily injections. These types of insulin are designed to mimic the way insulin is produced by the body, with appropriate injections of short-acting insulin with meals. It must be noted that several products have a premixed ratio of short-acting and intermediate-acting insulins (70%/30%, or 50%/50%). Based on your daily routines and meals, your doctor may prescribe you one of those to reduce the amount of daily injections and provide a better control of glucose after and between meals.

SPECIFIC DRUGS

Drug-Related Special Issues

The National Action Plan for Adverse Drug Event Prevention (ADE Action Plan) has identified diabetes medications among the main causes of common, preventable, and measurable adverse drug events. There are several important tips for safe treatment with oral drugs in DM. Below are summarized the main principles.

Metformin (Glucophage, others) is one the most effective oral medications for the treatment of type 2 DM. It is actually the only one clinically proven to reduce the incidence of damage to both small and large blood vessels (many other drugs have been shown to prevent only some of the complications, despite reducing blood glucose levels). If you were diagnosed with type 2 DM and do not have contraindications to *metformin*, it is most likely that you will be prescribed *metformin*.

TABLE 14.2 TYPES OF INSULINS USED FOR THE TREATMENT OF DIABETES MELLITUS

Insulin Type	Short or Long Acting	Onset	Peak*	Duration	Daily Frequency and Relation to Food
Lispro	Rapid acting	15 minutes	30–90 minutes	3–5 hours	2 or 3 times a day, depending on the regimen
Aspart	Rapid acting				
Regular	Short acting	30–60 minutes	2–4 hours	5–8 hours	
NPH	Intermediate acting	1–hour	8 hours	12–16 hours	Twice a day
Glargine (Lantus)	Long acting	1 hour	No peak	20 to 26 hours	Once daily
Detemir (Levemir)	Long acting				Once or twice daily

*Peak refers to the time it takes to achieve the peak (maximum) concentration of this type of insulin in the blood after injection.

The main conditions in which *metformin* should not be prescribed are impaired liver or kidney function because *metformin* is more likely to cause side effects when you have one of these conditions. It is also important to note that if you are taking *metformin*, you are at higher risk for kidney damage from contrast agents injected during diagnostic procedures like computer tomography (CT) or coronary angioplasty (used to open blocked coronary arteries supplying blood to the heart). *Metformin* needs to be discontinued before the procedure and restarted after kidney function tests show normal results. Make sure to ask about the use of contrast media in any diagnostic or interventional procedure you are planned to undergo, and whether and when you need to stop *metformin* before it. *Metformin* may reduce your vitamin B_{12} levels (you may need an under-the-tongue vitamin B_{12} supplement if vitamin B_{12} levels are below 200 picogram/mL). *Metformin* may also cause gastrointestinal symptoms—bloating, abdominal pain, diarrhea, or constipation. Usually taking the drug with food reduces the frequency of these side effects. Taking lower doses 3 times a day instead of higher doses twice a day, or sometimes just switching to another brand of *metformin*, may improve the side effects.

Sulfonylureas (glibenclamide/glyburide, glipizide). Once among the most common drugs used to treat DM, the use of sulfonylureas is declining. These are effective medication but have a few drawbacks. One is that they may cause hypoglycemia if you don't have a meal soon after taking them. The second issue is related to the mode of action of these drugs. Sulfonylureas stimulate the secretion of insulin from the pancreas. However, after taking sulfonylureas for about 5 years, the response of the pancreas to these drugs begins to decline in many patients. At a certain point, they are not able to stimulate enough insulin secretion to move glucose from the blood to tissues. Sulfonylureas such as *glyburide* may be an alternative to insulin in pregnant women with gestational diabetes mellitus.

Alpha-glucosidase inhibitors (*acarbose, miglitol*). These drugs need to be taken with the first bite of the meal, usually 2 to 3 times daily. High doses of these drugs may cause more side effects and are usually not associated with much improved effect on blood glucose. Alpha-glucosidase inhibitors slow down the absorption of glucose from the gastrointestinal tract and have been shown to improve HbA_{1c} in diabetic patients, but the effects are usually mild. Most common side effects include diarrhea, bloating, and abdominal pain. More than half of the patients do not tolerate these drugs because of side effects, but about 25 to 30% can benefit from long-term treatment, especially when added to other drugs such as *metformin* or *sulfonylurea*.

Dipeptidyl peptidase-4 inhibitors (*sitagliptin, linagliptin*) are available either alone or in fixed combination with *metformin* because clinical trials suggest they are more efficacious when combined.

Thiazolidinediones (*rosiglitazone* [Avandia], *pioglitazone* [Actos]) are to be taken once a day. *Rosiglitazone* started as a very promising drug, but long-term large studies have shown an increase in heart failure and myocardial infarction associated with the use of these drugs. The absolute risk is not very high but has to be considered carefully, especially in patients with any previous history or current heart disease. The first generation of these drugs caused liver issues in some patients; therefore, your prescriber may periodically order liver function tests if you are receiving thiazolidinediones.

The *incretin mimetics liraglutide* (Byetta), *exenatide* (Victoza), *dulaglutide* (Trulicity), and *albiglutide* (Tanzeum) all belong to the same class of drugs, but their administration regimens somewhat differ. *Liraglutide* is administered as daily self-injections under the skin, while the others are typically administered once a week as a self-injection under the skin. If you have a thyroid disease or are at high risk for thyroid cancer, your prescriber may decide to avoid these drugs or perform routine blood tests to ensure the drug is safe for you. Likewise, individuals who have a pancreas disease or are at high risk for pancreatitis or pancreatic cancer should avoid taking these drugs or should be under close monitoring.

The *sodium glucose cotransporter 2 (SGLT2) inhibitors canagliflozin* (Invokana), *dapagliflozin* (Farxiga), and *empagliflozin* (Jardiance) are currently the newest group of antidiabetic medications. Their efficacy seems to be moderate, and the initial data suggest they can help decrease the requirement of insulin in insulin-treated patients. On the other hand, the FDA recently warned that these medications may cause ketoacidosis (associated with only moderate increases in glucose blood levels). Several ongoing trials are aimed to help better understand the role of this group of medications in treating diabetes and address the safety concerns.

INSULIN

The general approach with insulin treatment targets both baseline glucose blood levels (i.e., between the meals) and also glucose levels after meals because naturally the carbohydrates we ingest cause an increase in blood sugar levels. In type 2 diabetes there is an ongoing debate on how early insulin treatment should be initiated if the initial treatment with oral drugs is unable to meet the targets of glucose and HbA_{1c} levels. There is no one secret formula, and the optimal approach with the safest and most effective regimen needs to be established between you and your physician.

If insulin treatment is initiated, it is important to understand whether the goal is to better control your between-meal glucose levels, the levels after meals, or both. Comprehensive training from a diabetes educator is extremely important for ensuring safe and effective use of insulin. Depending on the goals that were set with your physician, you may receive once-a-day or twice-a-day injections of long-acting insulin such as *glargine* or *detemir* to help with the basal insulin rate. Then, depending on your meal schedule, you may need two or three daily injections of short-acting insulins to control the after-meal glucose levels. Alternatively, you may be prescribed an injection of a mixed formulation (containing both short-acting and intermittently acting insulin) for two daily injections.

Certain individuals who rely more heavily on insulin, mainly people with type 1 diabetes, may choose to use insulin pumps. Insulin pumps include a fillable cartridge that contains short-acting insulin and is connected to a catheter that is placed under your skin. The pump is programmable and allows ongoing infusion of basal rate insulin; in addition, you have increased control in terms of when to press the button for additional doses and can decide on the insulin dose depending on the size of your meal.

The most important side effect of insulin is hypoglycemia, and it is typically the result of a mismatch between the amount of insulin that was received and the amount of food the person consumed. For example, if you injected your before-meal insulin dose and skipped the meal, insulin is likely to cause a drop of your blood glucose level from normal to low, instead of serving the purpose of reducing after-meal glucose levels from high to normal. Indeed, hypoglycemia has been identified as one of the most common and preventable adverse drug events for patients with diabetes. For example, between 2007 and 2009, among individuals older than 65 years, insulin was implicated in 14% of US emergent hospitalizations, and oral diabetes medications (discussed earlier) in 10.5% of emergent hospitalizations.

SPECIAL POPULATIONS

Children with diabetes typically suffer from type 1 DM, although type 2 diabetes in adolescents has been on the rise in the recent years. It is important to recommend early screening for children who have risk factors for diabetes, such as obesity, immediate relatives with type 2 diabetes, or early signs of insulin resistance such as polycystic ovaries in adolescent girls. Data have shown that parents who are themselves overweight tend to underestimate the diabetes risk associated with excess weight in their children and are likely to delay screening the children for DM. However, it is important to understand that early diagnosis of diabetes can be life-saving, and children with risk factors such as obesity or an immediate relative with diabetes need to be screened for the disease.

Pregnant women routinely undergo screening for gestational diabetes mellitus. Gestational diabetes increases the risk for undesired outcomes in pregnancy; therefore, it should be appropriately screened and addressed with diet modification, exercise, and, if appropriate, drug treatment.

IMPORTANT QUESTIONS TO ASK YOUR DOCTOR

It is challenging to provide an updated guidance on all the components of appropriate patient education in a short chapter. In addition, treatment and monitoring guidelines may change as new research becomes available. Nevertheless, it is important to ask your healthcare provider for updated educational materials on the following:

- *Diabetic ketoacidosis.* How can I prevent DKA? Do I have additional conditions that increase my risk for ketoacidosis? How will I know I am experiencing ketoacidosis? What should I do if I have symptoms of ketoacidosis?

- *Hypoglycemia.* You should ask the same set of questions as for DKA, only with replacing the word *ketoacidosis* with *hypoglycemia.*
- What are my blood glucose goals? What are my HbA$_{1c}$ goals?
- How and when should I measure my blood glucose levels at home? Is there a certain result (high or low) that necessitates seeking immediate medical care?
- What are the tests required to monitor the effect of diabetes on various organs—for example, eye exams, kidney tests, heart monitoring, neuropathy (sensory disturbance) tests? How frequently should each be performed, and what can I do to protect my various organs from diabetes-induced damage?

THINGS YOU CAN DO TO IMPROVE TREATMENT OUTCOMES

- Keep abreast of how to identify ketoacidosis and hypogly-cemia and have an action plan if these occur.
- Monitor blood glucose daily and record the results in a paper or electronic diary or spreadsheet (or use one of the health-care smartphone apps developed for that purpose). It will give you a good estimate of how well you are controlling your glucose and can help identify patterns of "bad days" or "bad weeks." You can then look at your routine in these "bad" periods and modify your lifestyle accordingly. There is no one-size-fits-all approach—each individual needs to find the balance between exercise, medication intake, and the fre-quency, ingredients, and size of their meals. And the optimal way to determine what works best for you is to record your

daily measurements and the daily routines and modify your lifestyle based on this objective feedback. Share this information with your physician or diabetes nurse or educator. Let them help you improve your routines for achieving better diabetes control.

- Being physically active and maintaining balanced diet can really make the difference. Activity like walking can also slow down some of the damage of diabetes to the nerve fibers in your feet and prevent *painful diabetic neuropathy*—one of the most common and bothersome complications of diabetes.
- Diabetic neuropathy may cause changes in your perception of temperature, touch, and pressure (in feet and sometimes in hands). As a consequence, you may not feel hot temperatures and are at increased risk for burn injury. In addition, your sensation of sharp objects is also reduced, so that you may not feel a pebble in a shoe or a minor cut. The immune system is weakened in diabetes, and wounds take a very long time to cure. Therefore, it is important that you inspect your feet daily for any cuts and wear appropriate shoes to avoid damage to your skin.

VALUABLE RESOURCES FOR ADDITIONAL EDUCATION ON DIABETES

American Diabetes Association: www.diabetes.org

Centers for Disease Control and Prevention: http://www.cdc.gov/diabetes/home

[15]

LET ME BREATHE!

Step-by-Step Asthma Management

Asthma is an inflammatory disease of the airways that causes episodes of wheezing, difficulty breathing, chest tightness, and coughing. These episodes are often associated with blockade (obstruction) of the airways, which can improve on its own or as a result of treatment. Asthma affects 7% of adults and 8.3% of the children in the United States and costs the US economy about $56 billion a year.

It is difficult to predict what exactly triggers an asthma attack in each individual. Some factors include an exposure to allergens, viruses, and indoor or outdoor pollutants. The exposure to an allergen usually causes an early allergic reaction that releases various inflammatory cells and molecules into the airway. This, in turn, leads to an inflammatory reaction within several hours. The result is narrowing of the airway and an increase in secretions into the airway, and this dual contribution limits the ability of air passage to and from the lungs.

Classically, asthma is characterized by difficulty in breathing associated with wheezing. However, the presentation may differ a lot among individuals, with persistent cough or chest tightness being the main complaint for some. In terms of frequency, asthma may present itself anywhere between occasional attacks with weeks or months of quiet periods (remission) all the way to daily symptoms. Cold and exercise can worsen or trigger the symptoms in some people, especially during allergen seasons such as the spring. For diagnosis, your doctor may perform several tests collectively called *spirometry* to determine certain measures of airway function, for example, to measure forced expiratory volume in 1 second (FEV_1), which is the volume of air one can exhale within 1 second. Spirometry measures can help both to determine the initial severity of asthma and to monitor treatment progress.

In addition to the presence of bothersome symptoms such as cough and wheezing, the harmful effects of asthma include the inability of the lungs to deliver a sufficient amount of oxygen to the blood because of restricted air passage through the inflamed airway. Severe asthma attacks can lead to impaired blood oxygenation and inability to remove carbon dioxide (CO_2) from the blood, resulting in a condition called *acidosis*. Severe untreated asthma can lead to respiratory failure and the need to connect the patient's airway to a mechanical ventilator machine to ensure proper oxygenation of vital organs such as the heart, brain, and kidneys.

TREATMENT GOALS

The main goals of treating asthma include the following:

1. Enable the person to maintaining normal activity levels, including exercise.
2. Maintain near normal pulmonary (lung) function.
3. Prevent symptoms such as coughing and breathlessness.

4. Prevent severe asthma attacks and the need for emergency department visits or hospital admissions.
5. Provide effective pharmacological treatment with minimal or no side effects.

TREATMENT APPROACH

The general treatment approach in asthma is tied to the severity of the disease. The idea is that the disease is divided into certain steps based on severity, and each step "deserves" a certain type of treatment, with the consideration of your individual symptoms and needs. Currently, the treatment approach includes the steps as outlined in Table 15.1. The table highlights the fact that for individuals with mild (or infrequent) symptoms, only treatment for symptoms is required, usually with no daily medications. If you have asthma symptoms more than twice a week, then it becomes important to get *daily* medication to prevent, or minimize, asthma attacks. This is one of the key concepts for successful control of asthma symptoms.

It is important to emphasize that Table 15.1 is only an example of the general treatment approach, and does not provide individual recommendations. The guidelines among North American and European (and other) organizations may differ, and recommendations are subject to change when new research evidence becomes available. Your healthcare provider will prescribe a treatment plan based on a similar guideline but may decide on a specific treatment approach considering your individual symptom pattern, response to therapy, other existing medical conditions, and medications.

TABLE 15.1 SEVERITY STEPS IN ASTHMA AND GENERAL TREATMENT APPROACH

Disease Severity/ Step	Frequency of Symptoms	Long-Term Control	Quick Relief
Step 1: Mild intermittent	Symptoms less than twice a week	No daily medications needed	Short-acting bronchodilator*
Step 2: Mild persistent	Symptoms more than twice a week but less than every day (asthma attacks may affect activity)	Usually one daily medication—either inhaled (e.g., low-dose steroid) or oral (e.g., *zafirlukast*)	Short-acting bronchodilator*
Step 3: Moderate persistent	Daily symptoms Daily use of inhaled short-acting bronchodilators* to control symptoms Exacerbations (flares) more than twice a week, may last days	Daily medication with either medium-dose inhaled steroid or a combination of low- to medium-dose steroid with long-acting bronchodilator* (frequently a single combo inhaler) If needed, your doctor may consider additional/alternative medications such as *zileuton* or *theophylline*	Short-acting bronchodilator*

| Step 4: Severe persistent | Continual symptoms Limited physical activity Frequent exacerbations | Daily medication with medium- to high-dose inhaled corticosteroids AND long-acting bronchodilator (inhaled or oral), often in addition to *omalizumab* or oral steroids, depending on asthma severity | Short-acting bronchodilator* |

*Bronchodilator is a medication that dilates, or widens, the bronchi (airway).

SPECIFIC DRUGS

As in other chapters, Table 15.2 summarizes the major classes of drugs used to treat asthma and presents how they are usually used, what is the mechanism by which they help control symptoms, and few possible tips that can help in using these drugs in a safer and more efficient way.

DRUG-RELATED SPECIAL ISSUES

It is important to know that there are several delivery systems to administer inhaled medications to the airway. Based on your age, motor coordination, and personal preference, your doctor can prescribe the medicine you require in the most convenient delivery system. One way to use asthma medications is through a nebulizer, where the liquid drug solution is added to a nebulizer container and you breathe the nebulized (vaporized) medication over several minutes. This is most commonly used in children and older adults who find it difficult to use inhalers. The more common delivery systems in adults are inhalers, which can be divided into a few types.

Metered-dose inhalers (MDIs) need to be shaken well before use because they contain the medicine mixed as a compressed gas. You should first *exhale*, then attach the mouthpiece of the inhaler to your mouth and *inhale at the same time* as pressing the container. This way you will ensure you are getting the maximum amount of medication to your airway.

Dry-powder inhalers (DPIs) usually need to be "loaded" before use. Per instruction on the specific DPI, the loading will include either twisting the inhaler or pressing a small lever. Hold it horizontally (parallel to the floor), unless specified otherwise by the manufacturer, and attach the mouthpiece to your mouth. Inhale rapidly.

TABLE 15.2 SUMMARY (AND EXAMPLES) OF MEDICATIONS FOR THE TREATMENT OF ASTHMA

Examples	Method of Administration	Drug Class	Mechanism	Administration Tips
Albuterol (ProAir, Ventolin), levalbuterol (Xopenex)	Inhalation (inhaler or nebulizer); can also be administered orally or intravenously	SABA—short-acting beta-2 agonist bronchodilators	These drugs activate beta-2 receptors in the airway smooth muscle and cause them to relax. The short-acting medications (SABA) act rapidly to relieve airways narrowing to improve breathlessness; the long-acting medications (LABA) work mainly by preventing airway narrowing for several hours	Follow your physician's orders in terms of number of puffs (if using inhaler) and the frequency. The use of SABA is usually based on symptom appearance
Formoterol (Foradil), Salmeterol (Serevent)	Inhalation (inhaler or nebulizer)	LABA—long-acting beta-2 agonist bronchodilators		The use of LABA is preventive—either daily or before exercise or allergen exposure
Budesonide (Pulmicort), fluticasone (Flovent)	Inhalation (inhaler)	Inhaled corticosteroids	Corticosteroids (or steroids) are anti-inflammatory drugs that help reduce the inflammation process in the airway for improving asthma symptoms	Unlike beta-2 agonists that work rapidly, corticosteroids work more slowly, and it may take hours or days to reach their maximum effect. Therefore, the primary use of inhaled steroids is not in treating an asthma attack but in the daily use for reducing the inflammation in the airways and preventing asthma symptoms

(continued)

TABLE 15.2 CONTINUED

Examples	Method of Administration	Drug Class	Mechanism	Administration Tips
Prednisone, prednisolone	Oral; intravenous (in severe cases)	Systemic corticosteroids		Oral corticosteroids may be administered daily (usually in low dose) for severe persistent asthma, or in short pulses (3–5 days) for asthma flares. Intravenous steroids may be administered in the hospital for treating severe asthma attacks
Theophylline	Oral; intravenous in emergencies	Xanthine Oxidase inhibitor	Theophylline relaxes airway smooth muscle cells by inhibiting a protein called xanthine oxidase. Theophylline may also have an anti-inflammatory effect	*Theophylline* may negatively interact with other medications (detailed further in Table 15.3). Because it is one of the "narrow therapeutic window" drugs (see Chapter 6), your doctor may request to measure its blood concentration from time to time. Some formulations of *theophylline* may be negatively affected by high-fat meals—ask your doctor or pharmacist whether the brand you have been prescribed is affected by meal. *Theophylline* is structurally similar to caffeine and shares some of its effects, such as diuretic

Drug	Route	Class/Mechanism type	Description
Nedocromil (Tilade, Alocril), cromolyn (Intal)	Inhalational	Mast cell stabilizer	Exact mechanism unknown, but both drugs inhibit the release of inflammatory molecules from immune cells	Both drugs are only effective by inhalation. These drugs do not have an immediate effect on relaxing the airways and therefore are of limited use in an acute asthma attack. They are more useful on a daily basis for prevention
Ipratropium (Atrovent), tiotropium (Spiriva)	Inhalational (inhaler or nebulizer); HandiHaler (a capsule with powder for inhalation)	Cholinergic antagonist (anticholinergic)	These drugs block the activation of acetylcholine receptors in the airway smooth muscle and cause muscle relaxation to increase the airway caliber (diameter)	Airway relaxation occurs not as fast as with SABA, but the effects last longer. Usually used as a nebulizer or inhaler (ipratropium). *Tiotropium* is delivered through a dry-powder inhalation system that releases the powder from a capsule
Zafirlukast (Accolate), montelukast (Singulair), zileuton (Zyflo)	Oral	Leukotriene modifiers	Leukotrienes are released from inflammatory cells and cause constriction of the airway, enhanced secretion, and additional inflammatory processes. These drugs reduce leukotriene-mediated inflammatory processes	Administered only orally. *Montelukast*—usually once a day, *zafirlukast*—twice a day. Absorption may be substantially affected by food—should be taken on an empty stomach (1 hour before or 2 hours after a meal) *Zileuton* is dosed 4 times a day. These drugs are not useful for treating acute asthma attacks. Used primarily for prevention in various degrees of persistent asthma

(continued)

TABLE 15.2 CONTINUED

Examples	Method of Administration	Drug Class	Mechanism	Administration Tips
Omalizumab (Xolair)	Subcutaneous (under the skin) injection every 2–4 weeks	Anti–immunoglobulin E (IgE) monoclonal antibody	By binding to human IgE, omalizumab reduces the inflammatory response to various allergens that cause IgE release and asthma worsening	*Omalizumab* is a biological product. The drug's dosing schedule is determined by IgE levels in the blood and your weight. It will usually be administered by your healthcare provider to monitor for any (rare) severe allergic reaction

You may not feel the actual powder, but most DPIs will have a little window with a number indicating the number of inhalations left. It is a good idea to follow the number to make sure you are not running out of medication.

If your inhaler contains a corticosteroid, it is highly advisable to *rinse your mouth* after the inhalation. Water can help flush any tiny pieces of powder that may attach to your mouth cavity and cause an irritation or stomatitis (canker sores).

Corticosteroid Tapering

With severe asthma attacks, you may be prescribed oral corticosteroids. In most outpatient cases, it would be a 3- to 5-day course of oral *prednisone* (or a similar drug). With this short-term use of corticosteroids, you could potentially get the same dose every day (e.g., 60 mg prednisone a day for 4 days). However, if the treatment is going to be prolonged, for more than 5 days, then a slow tapering is warranted by the end of the corticosteroid treatment. The tapering will usually mean gradual dose reduction, for example, from 60 mg/day to 45 mg/day, 30 mg/day, 25 mg/day, then 20, 15, and 10 mg/day.

This gradual tapering is important because the activity of many of our body's hormonal systems is based on a feedback loop. Our two adrenal glands, anatomically located one on top of each our kidneys, are organs that use cholesterol to produce cortisol, the body's main corticosteroid. In the feedback loop—when the cortisol concentration in our blood is too high, the adrenal glands do not release cortisol. The adrenals themselves do not respond to cortisol levels; rather, the feedback is mediated by another hormone, called adreno-corticotropic hormone (ACTH), that is released from the brain as a response to circulating corticosteroid levels. When someone gets a prolonged treatment with steroids, which causes a high level of steroids circulating in the blood, then ACTH will not be released, and the adrenal gland will temporarily stop *producing* cortisol. As long as you keep taking the prednisone, or a similar steroid, it will still serve the biological functions of cortisol produced by the adrenal glands because cortisol, prednisone, and other corticosteroids work on the same receptors. However, sudden discontinuation of the drug will cause a situation in which on one hand the adrenal gland is not producing enough cortisol (because the production was stopped by positive feedback of previous high concentrations in the blood), and on the other hand, you now don't have the exogenous steroid, prednisone. This will be similar to a condition in which the adrenal glands fail to function. Depending on the individual patient's condition and the duration (and dose) of treatment, the abrupt discontinuation of steroids can result in moderate symptoms such as fatigue, loss of appetite, nausea, diarrhea, and irritability, up to severe consequences such as drop in blood pressure, low blood levels of glucose, and high blood levels of potassium. My advice is: **never** discontinue oral corticosteroid treatment on your own. If for some reason you think the treatment is not appropriate for you, **always** consult your healthcare provider to discuss the optimal plan of corticosteroid tapering. If tapering is done correctly, the symptoms of adrenal failure can be **completely** prevented.

Use of Inhaled Beta Agonists

You should be aware that the use of short-acting beta-2 agonist (SABA) medications such as *albuterol* can cause tremor (shaking) and sometimes increased heart rate and headache. It is usually not recommended to use SABA frequently on a daily basis, and the maximal recommended dosage (for most SABAs) is two puffs 4 to 6 times a day. The prolonged use of beta-agonist inhalers, particularly without an inhaled steroid inhaler, has been associated with worse response to drugs during severe asthma attacks, and there has been a suggestion of increase in asthma-related deaths. However, it is important to highlight that the risk for death is extremely low, and the causality has not been established. The poorer outcomes may be associated with the drug itself, or with the fact that the patients who required very high doses simply had worse symptoms or were generally sicker. Newer studies are now conducted to understand this relationship better, but the current evidence suggests that if you have persistent asthma, a combination of a beta-2-agonist inhaler with a steroid inhaler provides more benefit than harm.

SABA may act on a certain transporter of ions in the muscle cell and cause potassium (K^+) ions to shift from the blood into the muscle cells. This may result in *hypokalemia,* a condition of reduced potassium in the blood. This is not common, but because potassium blood concentration is important for the activity of the heart, hypokalemia may result in cardiac rhythm disruption. If you have a heart condition, especially heart rhythm abnormalities (arrhythmia), and are chronically treated with SABA medications, you should consult your doctor about the need to periodically monitor your potassium levels.

Theophylline

Theophylline was one of the first and most common drugs used to treat asthma. Its use has dramatically decreased over the years, mainly because of its narrow therapeutic window, but some people still use it and benefit from it. Plasma concentrations of theophylline should be between 10 and 15 (up to 20) micrograms per milliliter (mcg/mL). The concentrations in different individuals, even with the same daily dose, are quite variable, and high plasma concentration (>30 mcg/mL) can increase the risk for seizures. Therefore, if you benefit from theophylline treatment and take it, it's a good idea to have periodic tests to measure its blood concentration to ensure safety. Do not switch brands of theophylline without proper consultation with your doctor and appropriate monitoring. In addition, there is a long list of drugs that potentially interact with theophylline. Table 15.3 lists some of the major ones, but this list is not exhaustive. If you are taking theophylline, always ask your doctor or the pharmacist about potential interactions each time you are treated with a new prescription or over-the-counter drug.

SPECIAL POPULATIONS

People Receiving Beta-Blockers

We discussed in length the use of beta-agonist drugs in asthma. Now there is an asthma-unrelated group of drugs called *beta-blockers* (e.g., *atenolol, propranolol,* and other drugs ending with *olol*), which are used for the treatment of high blood pressure (see Chapter 11) or different heart conditions such as heart failure. Some of these beta-blocker drugs (but not all of them) can worsen asthma symptoms because they can cause airway narrowing and diminish the effects of beta-agonist inhalers. If you have a heart condition or high blood pressure, together with asthma, make sure to discuss the use of beta-blockers with your physician to ensure a choice of a beta-1-selective blocker (e.g., *atenolol* or *metoprolol*), which can still address the heart condition but will have minimal effect on airway and asthma medications such as long-acting beta-2 agonists (LABAs) and SABAs.

Some eye drops for treating increased ocular pressure (*glaucoma*) also contain beta-blocker drugs. Despite being administered as eye drops, some of these drugs may worsen asthma symptoms. If you have asthma and also suffer from glaucoma or similar eye disease and

TABLE 15.3 POTENTIAL DRUG–DRUG INTERACTIONS
WITH THEOPHYLLINE

Drug	Used Usually for	Implication
Alcohol		Increase in theophylline blood concentration
Allopurinol	Gout	
Carbamazepine and phenytoin	Seizures	Decrease in theophylline blood concentration
Erythromycin, clarithromycin, ciprofloxacin	Antibiotics	Increase in theophylline blood concentration
Cimetidine	Gastric reflux or ulcers	
Estrogen		
Fluvoxamine	Antidepressant	
Mexiletine	Arrhythmia	
Benzodiazepines (diazepam, lorazepam)	Treatment of anxiety	Larger antianxiety medication doses may be required
Zafirlukast and zileuton	Asthma	Both can increase theophylline blood concentration; caution is required if these are co-prescribed for asthma management

use eye drops, consult with your physician or pharmacist to prevent a negative effect of beta-blocker eye drops on your asthma.

Children

Children are a very large population among asthma sufferers, and although this is beyond the scope of this chapter, age-adjusted guidelines are available for treating asthmatic children. These guidelines also include steps based on persistence and severity of the condition, although the stepwise approach somewhat differs from the adult approach. Children with persistent asthma, mainly the ones with a more severe disease, may require long-term use of inhaled corticosteroids to control their symptoms, a treatment that has been concerning many parents (and pediatricians). The main concern has been with the risk for growth inhibition and impaired bone mineral density in these children. I would like to emphasize that inhaled corticosteroids are only partially absorbed into the bloodstream. Therefore, their side effects are by far less frequent than with long-term treatment with oral or injectable steroids. This is not to say that there is absolutely no risk with inhaled corticosteroids, but it is important to know that the effect of steroids on growth is dose-dependent. Research studies have shown that children treated with low-to-medium doses of daily inhaled corticosteroids do not differ in height from their counterparts who were not treated with steroids. Children with more severe asthma, who require long-term high doses of inhaled corticosteroids, are at higher risk for impaired growth and lower bone mineral density. With that said, the individual risk is variable, and many children on high-dose inhaled steroids are doing fine. The key, I believe, is in appropriate monitoring. If a child receives a moderate to high dose of inhaled corticosteroids on a chronic basis, it is highly advisable to monitor the child's height on standard growth curves every 3 to

6 months and ask your child's doctor if yearly bone mineral density tests are required.

IMPORTANT QUESTIONS TO ASK YOUR DOCTOR

- What is the current severity of my asthma?
- What are the treatment goals for me?
- What is my goal FEV_1?
- Which are the daily medications I need to use for prevention of asthma attacks, and which should I use for treating an acute asthma attack?
- What medication side effects should I expect, and which I should be concerned with?

THINGS YOU CAN DO TO IMPROVE TREATMENT OUTCOMES

Monitor your symptoms. Remember, *if you cannot measure it, you cannot improve it.* It is advisable to record the weekly frequency of symptoms in order to have a good estimate of how well your asthma symptoms are controlled. This can be done in a paper, electronic, or mobile app diary, whichever is more convenient for you. It can help optimize medication doses, identify whether certain interventions help, and if so, how much they help, but also identify triggers that worsen the frequency of asthma attacks. This valuable information can help you and your doctor make more intelligent decisions for safely preventing and treating your asthma. *Spirometry* can provide an additional quantitative measure of treatment efficacy, beyond registering symptom frequency. Ask your doctor whether you should use these measures at home (or only at office visits) to monitor your asthma better and help prevent emergency department visits.

Stick to your prescribed medication regimen. If your symptoms have been controlled well with medications, don't stop taking them assuming your asthma is better now. Discuss with your doctor whether it may be appropriate to "step down" your drug regimen and how to do so safely.

Control your weight. Obese people are 50% more likely to suffer from asthma symptoms. If your weight is excessive, participating in healthy nutrition and weigh loss program can also help you control your asthma, in addition to the added benefits of weight reduction on general health.

Know and prevent side effects. Try to identify triggers to asthma attacks (allergens, exercise, and weather) and either avoid these triggers or use pre-exposure prophylaxis with appropriate medications. For example, for exercise-induced asthma, LABAs inhaled before exercise can be beneficial. In children with seasonal allergies, sometimes pretreatment with drugs such as *omalizumab* can reduce exacerbations.

VALUABLE RESOURCES FOR ADDITIONAL EDUCATION ON ASTHMA

Centers for Disease Control and Prevention: http://www.cdc.gov/asthma/

National Heart, Lung, and Blood Institute: http://www.nhlbi.nih.gov/health/health-topics/topics/asthma

[16]

EPILEPSY

Understand Your Drugs to Stop the Seizures

Approximately one of every 25 people will develop epilepsy at some point in their lifetime, and somewhere between 3 and 3.5 million people currently live with epilepsy in the United States. In two thirds of these people, the seizures are controlled with treatment, but about one third live with uncontrolled seizures.

A seizure is defined as the clinical manifestation of excessive (and out of sync) activity of nerve cells (neurons) in the brain. Although *epilepsy* is a term that covers a variety of "seizure disorders," it is important to understand that not every seizure is epilepsy. Seizures may occur for different reasons: imbalance of electrolytes (salts) in the body, fever, withdrawal from drugs or alcohol, or sleep deprivation, to name a few. In these isolated episodes, it is assumed that after these abnormalities are corrected, the person will not have more seizures. Epilepsy, as opposed to these isolated seizures, will be diagnosed when a patient has repeated (recurrent) seizures, not provoked by abnormalities as described previously. Many think of epilepsy as a disease in which people convulse, lose consciousness, have foam coming out of their mouth, and swallow their tongue. While this severe picture describes the condition of a "generalized tonic-clonic seizure" (except the fact that people cannot swallow their tongue), this is only one type of epilepsy, among a group of a dozen different subtypes of seizure disorders.

The exact mechanism for why seizures occur is not well understood. The patterns of abnormal electrical activity in brain cells have been studied, and it is often possible to see characteristic findings in the brain's electrical activity on an electroencephalogram (EEG), a common test that every patient with suspected epilepsy is likely to undergo. However, what exactly triggers this abnormal electrical activity in the various types of seizure disorders is yet unclear. In some people the seizures tend to occur after certain events such as flashing lights or loud music, or are associated with physiological or psychological factors such as intense exercise, strong emotions, or stress. In some cases of diagnosed epilepsy, there is an identifiable cause such as head trauma, brain tumor, or stroke; however, in the majority of individuals the reason for seizures remains unknown.

In this chapter, I will briefly summarize the different types of epilepsy and focus on the specifics of safe and effective medication management. The reason for describing the various types of seizures (summarized in Table 16.1) is that each type of seizure disorder may be associated with different risks and managed with different medications, which, in turn, have very different safety profiles.

Partial (focal) seizures are divided into two gross categories, depending on whether they occur with or without impairment of consciousness. These seem to occur within certain brain regions and do not involve the whole brain, although in some cases a focal seizure can develop into a generalized seizure (discussed in the next paragraph). The symptoms of focal seizures vary from one person to another and depend on the location in which the seizure originated in the brain. As a result, the seizure may begin as a sensation of flashing lights or movements of the face, arm, or a leg. For a given individual, the pattern of partial (focal) seizures will be similar each time because typically the same brain region is involved.

TABLE 16.1 TYPES OF SEIZURES

Epilepsy (Seizure Disorders)

Partial (Focal) Seizures		Generalized Seizures
Partial seizures without impairment of consciousness	Partial seizures with impairment of consciousness	Generalized tonic-clonic seizures (flexion of limbs, followed by clonic [jerking] movements, loss of consciousness, gradual return to awareness within 15–30 minutes)
Motor expressions such as jerking of one limb, or sensory expressions such as foul odor or visual disturbance. Patients do not lose awareness and can respond to their environment throughout the seizure	Impaired consciousness can be accompanied by a variety of abnormal motor and sensory expressions, often with automatic behaviors such as lip smacking, doing and undoing buttons, or wandering. Patients may experience aura	Absence seizures (occur mainly in children), are characterized by sudden interruption of awareness, followed by a fixed stare; they may be accompanied by aforementioned movements Myoclonic, tonic, and atonic seizures (each is different), are characterized by sudden loss of muscle tone, jerking movements, or other partial muscle expressions of tonic-clonic seizures

In contrast to focal seizures, *generalized seizures* appear to originate in all regions of the brain cortex simultaneously. Absence seizures and generalized tonic-clonic seizures are common types of generalized seizures, along with clonic, myoclonic, tonic, and atonic seizures.

Absence seizures (also called *petit mal*) usually occur during childhood and typically last between 5 and 10 seconds. They frequently occur in clusters and may take place dozens or even hundreds of times a day. Absence seizures cause sudden staring with impaired consciousness. If an absence seizure lasts for 10 seconds or more, then eye blinking and lip smacking may also appear.

A *generalized tonic-clonic seizure* (also called *grand mal* seizure, or convulsion) is the most dramatic type of seizure. It begins with a sudden loss of consciousness, often in association with a scream or shriek. All of the muscles of the arms and legs, as well as the chest and the back, become stiff. After approximately 1 minute, the muscles begin to jerk and twitch for an additional 1 to 2 minutes. During this clonic (twitching) phase, the tongue can be bitten.

Myoclonic seizures (literally—*muscle twitching* seizures) consist of sudden, brief muscle contractions that may occur as a single contraction or in clusters and that can affect any group of muscles, although typically the arms are affected. Consciousness is usually not impaired.

Tonic seizures cause sudden muscle stiffening, often associated with impaired consciousness and falling to the ground.

Atonic seizures (also known as drop seizures) produce the opposite effect of tonic seizures: a sudden loss of control of the muscles, particularly of the legs, that results in collapsing to the ground and possible injuries.

During seizures with impairment of consciousness, the person may appear to be awake but is not in contact with others in the environment and does not respond normally to instructions or questions.

People often seem to stare into space and either remain motionless or engage in repetitive behaviors, called *automatisms*, such as facial grimacing, gesturing, chewing, lip smacking, snapping fingers, repeating words or phrases, walking, running, or undressing. It is important not to try to physically restrain people during these seizures because they may become hostile or aggressive. The better way is to try to comfort the person during these seizures.

Many people with epilepsy do not have a warning when their seizures start. Instead, they suddenly lose consciousness, which they may describe as blacking out, when the part of the brain cortex that controls memory is disrupted by the seizure. Afterward, particularly after generalized tonic-clonic seizure, the individual enters the *postictal* phase, often characterized by sleepiness, confusion, and headache for up to several hours. The person typically has no memory of what took place during the seizure. Some people may have a sort of a warning sign before the seizure, which is called *aura*. Aura is a perceptual disturbance, which often manifests as the perception of a strange light, an unpleasant smell, or confusing thoughts or experiences. Although people don't remember their experience of the seizure itself, they may remember the aura that preceded it.

TREATMENT GOALS

The main treatment goal in epilepsy is to completely control the seizures in order to allow normal or near-normal quality of life.

TREATMENT APPROACH

Antiepileptic drugs are the mainstay of epilepsy treatment. The choice of the specific antiepileptic drug (or their combination) will be based on the type of seizures and the person's age, gender, existing medical conditions, other medications, and individual preferences based on potential drug side effects. The additional treatment goals, beyond maximizing seizure control, should also be chosen on an individual basis.

Treating epilepsy is a challenging task. There are a variety of drugs that work well, but unfortunately, most antiepileptic drugs come with a risk for serious side effects. Some of these drugs would not be considered safe if they were to be prescribed for other milder, less dangerous diseases. However, because epilepsy is a condition that is associated by a higher mortality (1.5 to 3 times higher than in general population), in addition to potential injuries associated with broken bones, concussions, and bleeding, the individual consideration of risks versus benefits is of high importance. This risk assessment should be performed with the treating neurologist, and I believe no textbook information can, or should, substitute proper clinical judgment in such cases.

The good news is that about 70% of people with epilepsy can be maintained effectively on a single antiepileptic drug. The bad news is that about 60% of individuals with epilepsy don't comply with their treatment, and the **lack of compliance** is the **most common** reason that epilepsy treatments fail. It's difficult to blame the patients for not being compliant because many of these drugs have frequent and bothersome side effects and people are not very happy to take them. However, with a responsible approach to adherence, there is an opportunity and a reasonable chance to obtain close to normal quality of life with epilepsy.

Treatment of epilepsy is sometimes a lifelong journey. However, a seizure-free period of 2 to 4 years is usually a very good prognostic factor, especially when it is accompanied with normal EEG findings. Actually, after a 2- to 5-year seizure-free period, your neurologist might try to gradually reduce the dose of your antiepileptic drug(s), and in some cases the treatment can be stopped.

SPECIFIC DRUGS

I will not be attempting to assign the various antiepileptic drugs by type of seizures they can help control because your doctor will help you choose the appropriate drug (or combination of drugs) based on your conditions and preferences. Without getting too much into the mechanisms, all antiepileptic drugs work by reducing hyperactivity of nerve cells (neurons) in the brain. There is always a difference in voltage between the inside of a neuron and outside its membrane. For neurons to become activated and transmit electrical signals, this difference in voltage needs to change. This occurs by shifting electrolytes, which are either positively charged ions (e.g., sodium, potassium and calcium) or negatively charged ions (e.g., chlorine) in or out of cells. In most neurons relevant to this chapter, higher positive charge (more positive ions and/or less negative ions) inside the cell would translate into excessive electrical activity. Therefore, antiepileptic drugs typically control the hyperactivity of neurons in the brain by either blocking channels whose activity will increase the concentration of positively charged ions in the cell, or enhancing the activity of channels (e.g., the gamma-aminobutyric acid [GABA] channel) whose activity would increase concentration of negatively charged ions in the cell.

Table 16.2 lists the most commonly used drugs for treating epilepsy, briefly describes the types of epilepsy they are most useful in, and suggests some tips on administration, need for blood concentration monitoring, and potential for drug interactions.

TABLE 16.2 COMMON ANTIEPILEPTIC DRUGS

Drug/Drug Class (and Examples)	Commonly Used in the Following Types of Seizures	Important to Monitor Blood (Plasma) Levels?	Subject to Numerous Drug Interactions?
Carbamazepine (Tegretol, others) and oxcarbazepine (Trileptal)	Generalized tonic-clonic seizures, partial seizures	Not necessary, but may be advised with carbamazepine if seizures are not well-controlled	Yes, major. Main consequence: reduced blood concentration (and effectiveness) of other drugs. Carbamazepine is a stronger inducer of liver enzymes than oxcarbazepine (higher risk for interactions with carbamazepine)
Phenytoin (Dilantin)	Generalized tonic-clonic seizures, partial seizures	Yes, routinely. Phenytoin blood concentration should be within 10–20 mcg/mL	Yes, major. Main consequence: reduced blood concentration (and effectiveness) of other drugs
Valproate, valproic acid (Depakote, others)	Generalized tonic-clonic seizures, partial seizures, absence seizures, myoclonic seizures	Yes, routinely. Valproate blood concentrations should be within 50–100 mcg/mL	Yes, major. A variety of mechanisms—in most cases, increased toxicity of valproate. Valproate can also increase toxicity of other drugs
Lamotrigine (Lamictal)	Generalized tonic-clonic seizures, partial seizures, myoclonic seizures	Typically not necessary	Yes, moderate. Main outcome: lamotrigine blood concentrations affected

TABLE 16.2 CONTINUED

Drug/Drug Class (and Examples)	Commonly Used in the Following Types of Seizures	Important to Monitor Blood (Plasma) Levels?	Subject to Numerous Drug Interactions?
Topiramate (Topamax)	Generalized tonic-clonic seizures, partial seizures	No	Yes, moderate. Main consequence: topiramate is an inducer of liver enzymes (may affect other drugs), but the effect is less significant than with carbamazepine or phenytoin
Lacosamide (Vimpat)	Partial seizures	No	Only a few known
Ethosuximide (Zarontin)	Absence seizures	May be required	Yes, moderate. Ethosuximide primarily affected
Gabapentin (Neurontin) and pregabalin (Lyrica)	Partial seizures, secondary generalized seizures	No	Almost none. Avoid taking with antacids
Levetiracetam (Keppra)	Generalized tonic-clonic seizures, partial seizures, myoclonic seizures	No	Only a few known. Primarily with other antiepileptics such as carbamazepine and phenytoin. Interacts with methotrexate (used for immunosuppression)

(*continued*)

TABLE 16.2 CONTINUED

Drug/Drug Class (and Examples)	Commonly Used in the Following Types of Seizures	Important to Monitor Blood (Plasma) Levels?	Subject to Numerous Drug Interactions?
Benzodiazepines such as clonazepam (Klonopin) and clobazam (Frisium, Onfi) for oral treatment, diazepam and lorazepam for intravenous use	Focal, myoclonic seizures, usually used to stop a seizure.	No	Yes, major. Main consequence: benzodiazepines are affected by other drugs or can worsen sleepiness with other sedating drugs
Barbiturates Phenobarbital (Luminal), Primidone (Mysoline)	Generalized tonic-clonic seizures, partial seizures; often used as an injection to stop a seizure	Yes (phenobarbital)	Yes, major. Main consequence: reduced blood concentration (and effectiveness) of other drugs through liver enzyme induction
Tiagabine (Gabitril)	Partial seizures	May be required	Yes, moderate. Main consequence: tiagabine blood concentrations are affected by other drugs
Vigabatrin (Sabril)	Refractory focal epilepsy	No	Only a few known. Primarily with other antiepileptics such as carbamazepine and phenytoin

TABLE 16.2 CONTINUED

Drug/Drug Class (and Examples)	Commonly Used in the Following Types of Seizures	Important to Monitor Blood (Plasma) Levels?	Subject to Numerous Drug Interactions?
Felbamate (Felbatol)	Myoclonic seizures, usually restricted to patients with refractory seizures, because of potentially severe side effects	No	Yes, major. Main consequences: risk for arrhythmias with other drugs that affect heart rhythm. May increase or decrease the metabolism of other drugs

DRUG-RELATED SPECIAL ISSUES

Generally, antiepileptic drugs, as a class, are considered to have the most drug–drug interactions. It would be impossible to list all the possible interactions, but the likelihood and severity are briefly outlined in Table 16.2. You can refer to this table if you are taking one of these drugs, and make sure you check with a reliable health-care provider **every time** a new drug is prescribed to you, or when you are thinking of taking an over-the-counter drug or a herbal supplement. It is important to remember that interactions with antiepileptic drugs can occur in both directions: they can influence other drugs (by decreasing their effect or increasing their toxicity), and certain drugs can affect antiepileptic drugs by increasing their toxicity or reducing their effect.

In addition, treatment with antiepileptic drugs can increase the incidence of suicidal thoughts. The absolute risk is not very high (approximately one case of suicidal thinking for every 530 patients treated), but it is higher than in patients who are not treated with anti-epileptic drugs. People should be aware of this risk and seek medical care if such thoughts or behaviors occur, especially if they had been suffering from depression or having depressive symptoms in the past.

In general, abrupt discontinuation of antiepileptic medication is not recommended because it may trigger seizures. If a decision has been made to stop a certain drug, you should consult with your physician about the appropriate regimen for gradual tapering of the drug over several days or weeks.

I cannot stress enough the importance of adherence to your treatment regimen. Most antiepileptic drugs need to maintain a certain concentration in the brain (and therefore in the blood) to prevent neuronal hyperactivity. Once the concentrations fall below a certain threshold, you are not protected from the next seizure. On the other hand, most antiepileptic drugs have unpleasant side effects (e.g., drowsiness, nausea, confusion, tremors, and loss of balance), especially if the concentration in the blood is too high. Unlike many other drugs that are not as sensitive to fluctuations, such as occasional missed doses, the adherence is of EXTREME importance in epilepsy. Yes, it is difficult to remember and take all the drugs properly and on time. Yes, it requires an enormous effort on your behalf. But in most cases in which proper adherence is maintained, it can make all the difference in achieving your treatment goals. Use whatever tricks you can to take your medications on time: use a smartphone app, alarm clocks, sticky notes with reminders, or notes on your refrigerator or the bathroom mirror or reward yourself with something positive (like turning on your favorite song or looking at your favorite photograph) every time you take your medications on time—whatever works for you. Don't skip doses, and don't skip the required periodic blood tests.

I mentioned that many antiepileptic drugs are associated with frequent side effects or toxicities. The list is long, but the subsequent sections summarize the important drug-specific side effects to be aware of, to prevent life-threatening situations.

Carbamazepine (Tegretol, Others) and Oxcarbazepine (Trileptal)

Doses should be increased gradually to minimize side effects such as nausea and drowsiness. *Carbamazepine* may cause elevation of liver enzymes, but in most cases it is mild. Among more serious problems are potential effects on white blood cells; your physician is likely to order periodic blood tests to monitor for these effects. Serious skin reactions may occur; in any case of rash or unusual skin reactions, seek immediate medical care. *Carbamazepine* has the ability to induce its own metabolism, therefore, some of its side effects (and plasma levels) will be reduced within 2 to 4 weeks of therapy initiation or dose increase. Do not chew or brake sustained-release carbamazepine tablets. If you are taking *carbamazepine* oral liquid (suspension), schedule it between 1 and 2 hours before taking other liquid medications. Do not switch brands of *carbamazepine* without proper consultation with your doctor and without appropriate monitoring.

Oxcarbazepine profile is somewhat similar to carbamazepine, although it has less substantial interactions, and it has a somewhat safer side-effect profile. As a side note, *oxcarbazepine* and *carbamazepine* are sometimes used for the treatment of a facial pain condition called *trigeminal neuralgia* (*tic douloureux*).

Phenytoin (Dilantin, Others)

Phenytoin is an effective antiepileptic drug. Usually, the desired blood concentration in adults is around 15 mcg/mL, with concentration in the range of 5 to 20 mcg/mL usually providing good epilepsy control without toxicity. *Phenytoin* has very unusual pharmacokinetics (mainly its elimination process), and sometimes small increases in its dose can result in disproportionately high concentrations in the blood and, accordingly, in side effects. Signs of *phenytoin* toxicity, associated with high blood concentration, are visual disturbances, sleepiness, nausea and vomiting, and uncontrolled body movements. Other side effects include heart rhythm changes, thickening of the gums, and rash.

Phenytoin is available in various salt forms, so the dose might change a little if switching from one product to another. Do not switch brands without proper consultation with your doctor and without appropriate monitoring.

Valproate (Valproic Acid) (Depakote, Others)

Valproate is a very effective antiepileptic. Because *valproate* carries a risk for liver failure and has a potential effect on platelets, you should be attentive to side effects such as appearance of weakness, jaundice (skin turning yellow), vomiting, persistent bleeding, or bruising. Tremor (shaking) and excessive sleepiness might be signs of higher than normal (toxic) blood concentrations. Other side effects may include swelling of the feet or hands, dizziness, intestinal symptoms, visual disturbances, rash, and hair loss. Do not crush or chew sustained-release tablets.

Some antibiotics administered intravenously in the hospital setting can almost completely neutralize the effect of *valproate* by reducing its blood concentrations. If your seizures are treated with valproate and you happen to be hospitalized for an infection, make sure your physicians are aware of your *valproate* treatment, especially if you are treated with an antibiotic that ends with *penem* (e.g., *meropenem*).

Lamotrigine (Lamictal, Others)

Serious skin reactions (at a rate of 3 of 1000 patients) may occur with *lamotrigine*, usually within 8 weeks of treatment initiation. To minimize this effect, *lamotrigine* will usually be initiated at low doses and increased gradually every 1 to 2 weeks. Visual disturbance are quite common, as are nausea and dizziness.

Topiramate (Topamax)

Drink plenty of fluids while taking *topiramate* because the drug may increase the risk for kidney stones. Side effects may include cognitive problems (mainly with speech and memory), nervousness, tremor, visual disturbances, weight loss, and various gastrointestinal symptoms. *Topiramate* dose is usually increased gradually, with weekly dose increments, to allow adjustment to side effects. As a side note, *topiramate* is also quite frequently used for migraine headache prevention.

Lacosamide (Vimpat)

Patients with heart disease and heart rhythm abnormalities treated with *lacosamide* are at higher risk for arrhythmias. It is recommended to obtain baseline electrocardiogram (ECG) and follow up to ensure lack of heart toxicity. In addition, *lacosamide* may cause nausea, dizziness, and visual disturbances. Most of the drug is excreted by the kidney—patients with kidney disease may need closer monitoring and dose adjustment.

Ethosuximide (Zarontin)

Severe skin reactions may occur with *ethosuximide*. Nausea and upset stomach are among the most common side effects. *Ethosuximide* may cause blood cell abnormalities, such that periodic blood count monitoring is recommended. Be attentive to side effects such as sore throat, general malaise, and easy bruising because they may indicate changes in blood cell counts and require additional tests.

Gabapentin (Neurontin, Others) and Pregabalin (Lyrica)

Neither of these two drugs is usually used alone to treat epilepsy; they are typically add-on options to improve seizure control. Both *gabapentin* and *pregabalin* are quite safe compared with other antiepileptic drugs, have very few drug interactions, and do not require blood concentration monitoring. Both may cause dizziness, sleepiness, and swelling of the feet. These two drugs are more frequently used for the treatment of nerve injury–related pain (see Chapter 18).

Levetiracetam (Keppra)

Levetiracetam is also considered one of the safest antiepileptic drugs, although serious skin reactions may occur as well as blood cell abnormalities. *Levetiracetam* may decrease bone mineral density over time, so monitoring may be appropriate.

Benzodiazepines, Primarily Clonazepam (Klonopin) and Clobazam (Frisium, Onfi)

Benzodiazepines are among the only few antiepileptic drugs that may cause dependence on continued use. Dependence does not mean addiction, but abrupt stopping, in addition to increasing the risk for seizures, may cause withdrawal symptoms. Doses of benzodiazepines should be increased slowly; these are also antianxiety medications and can cause somnolence. Avoid alcohol if you are treated with these medications. Benzodiazepines are associated with substantially lower rates of severe skin reactions, effects on blood cells, and liver failure compared with other antiepileptic drugs. Their use with opioid analgesics such as morphine or oxycodone increases the risk for respiratory failure.

Barbiturates, Primarily Phenobarbital (Luminal) and Primidone (Mysoline)

Barbiturates can cause excessive sleepiness and reduce alertness. They have fewer effects on blood cell counts compared with other antiepileptic drugs. Alcohol or other nervous system depressant drugs should be avoided. *Phenobarbital* has substantial interactions with other drugs, including oral contraceptives. It reduces oral contraceptive efficacy by inducing liver and gut enzymes.

Tiagabine (Gabitril)

Tiagabine may cause generalized weakness, swelling of the extremities, high blood pressure, and heart rhythm abnormalities. Hair loss and visual changes have also been reported as well as excessive bleeding during menstrual cycle in women. Dose reduction may be necessary in people with liver disease.

Vigabatrin (Sabril)

Vigabatrin may cause potentially serious visual field effects, including vision loss; the risk increases with dose and treatment duration. Therefore, its use is quite restricted.

Felbamate (Felbatol)

Felbamate may cause serious, sometimes fatal, suppression of blood cell production in the bone marrow and liver failure. These side effects are rare, but similarly to *vigabatrin*, its use is restricted to special circumstances.

SPECIAL POPULATIONS

Women Who Are Pregnant or Are Planning Pregnancy

Antiepileptic drugs can increase the risk for congenital abnormalities in the fetus, especially if the exposure occurred in the first trimester (weeks 1 to 12) of pregnancy. As we discussed in Chapter 10, there is a 2 to 4% chance in the general population that a child is born with some congenital abnormality, but exposure to antiepileptic drugs can increase this risk. On the other hand, untreated epilepsy during the pregnancy bears significant risks to the developing fetus as well; therefore, it is important that you and your doctor thoroughly discuss the risks and the benefits of treatment **before** pregnancy.

Levetiracetam and *lamotrigine* are considered relatively safe during pregnancy. Valproate, on the other hand (especially at high doses), is considered to carry the highest risk. The dose of the antiepileptic drug may also be very important. For example, a *valproate* dose of below 1000 mg/day is reported to increase the risk for birth abnormalities to 5%, but a dose above 1000 mg/day may increases the risk to 9%. In general, it is recommended to control epilepsy with a single drug and the lowest possible dose before pregnancy. Addition of folic acid, started before pregnancy, at around 4 mg daily dose, can reduce the risk for certain birth malformations. During pregnancy, several physiological parameters change (e.g., amount of water in the body);

therefore, some adjustment in the drug dosages might be necessary. The **most important** recommendation to women with epilepsy is to plan their pregnancy and to consult a neurologist and obstetrician ahead of time about choosing the optimal treatment approach.

Women Who Are Using Contraception

Women of childbearing age who are treated with (most) antiepileptic drugs will be required to use a double-barrier method (e.g., an oral contraceptive pill plus a condom) or an oral contraceptive with a relatively high dose of hormones. As outlined in Table 16.2, many antiepileptic drugs can induce cytochrome P-450 (CYP) enzymes in the liver, which, among other things, break down estrogens. This enzymatic induction, therefore, will reduce the amount of circulating hormones in the blood and impair the effectiveness of the oral contraceptive. Adding insult to injury, beyond the undesired pregnancy in this case, the fetus will be also exposed to the antiepileptic drug in first trimester, which, as we discussed in the previous paragraph, is an undesirable outcome on its own.

IMPORTANT QUESTIONS TO ASK YOUR DOCTOR

- What are the serious side effects of each of my drugs, and how can I identify them as soon as possible?
- What is the potential of drug interactions with my current drugs, and what kind of other medications should I be concerned with?
- Do I need periodic blood tests for either monitoring the concentrations of my antiepileptic drugs in blood or monitoring potential toxicities?

THINGS YOU CAN DO TO IMPROVE TREATMENT OUTCOMES

- Stick to your treatment. The balance between efficacy and toxicity in antiepileptic drugs is particularly delicate. It's easy to lose this balance by missing doses, changing medication brands, or adding or stopping other medications. If you and your doctor have found a drug that controls your seizures well without substantial side effects, try to do your absolute best, day after day, to faithfully stick to the treatment.

- If you develop sudden fever or fatigue, sometimes associated with skin reactions, you should notify your doctor immediately because it may be a sign of your drug affecting your blood cells.

- Always keep an updated list of your antiepileptic medications and provide it to **every** provider who prescribes you a new medicine.

- Some medications may cause or worsen seizures. It is important to avoid these (if possible) or be minded that an adjustment in the dose of your antiepileptic drugs may be necessary. Among these drugs are certain antibiotics, a number of antidepressant medications, antipsychotic medications, and analgesics like tramadol. Alcohol and certain illicit drugs, such as amphetamines and cocaine, can substantially increase the risk for seizures and must be avoided.

VALUABLE RESOURCES FOR ADDITIONAL EDUCATION ON EPILEPSY

National Institutes of Neurological Disorders and Stroke: https://www.ninds.nih.gov/Disorders/All-Disorders/Epilepsy-Information-Page

Epilepsy Foundation: http://www.epilepsy.com/learn/about-epilepsy-basics

[17]

HOPING FOR A BETTER DAY

Treating Depression

Depression is a common condition, with several current theories behind what causes it. Among the leading thoughts is that depression is a neurobiological disease caused by an imbalance of certain molecules (neurotransmitters) in the brain, mainly of serotonin. In addition to the neurotransmitter imbalance, a tendency of negative thinking and low self-esteem, presence of other illnesses (diabetes, chronic pain, or heart disease), situational factors such as difficult life events, and genetic factors may all contribute. There are several subtypes of depression, with major depressive disorder (also called *unipolar depressive disorder*) being the main one. The term unipolar is used to distinguish it from *bipolar* disorders, otherwise called manic-depressive disorder.

The symptoms that are characteristic of major depression, which are also used for diagnosing the disorder, occur on a (nearly) daily basis and include some of the following:

1. Depressed mood most of the day
2. Loss of interest or pleasure in most or all activities
3. Too much or too little sleep
4. Significant changes in weight or appetite

5. Slowing down of movements and speech (or in some cases, uncontrolled and purposeless movements) that is observable by others
6. Fatigue or low energy
7. Decreased ability to concentrate, think, or make decisions
8. Thoughts of worthlessness or excessive or inappropriate guilt
9. Repeated thoughts of death or suicidal thoughts, or a suicide attempt

When these symptoms are not caused by drugs (legal or illicit) or by another medical condition and they result in significant distress or anxiety or negatively affect behavior and social activities, it is likely that the person is suffering from a depressive disorder, although an accurate diagnosis requires an evaluation by a trained healthcare professional such as a psychiatrist or a psychologist.

Between 8.5 and 10% of people in the United States and Europe have depression, and about 20% of Americans and 14% of Europeans will meet depression criteria at least once during their lifetime. These numbers show that depression is not necessarily a permanent disorder because it may sometimes improve over time or can be effectively treated. Women are almost twice as likely to experience depression compared with men, although the reason for this difference is unclear. Depression is associated with high mortality by suicide, which is the number 11 cause of death in the United States, accounting for 30,000 deaths per year (more than 80 every day). Beyond the high mortality rate, depression causes substantial disability and loss of productivity. The estimated costs related to depression and related disorders to the US society range between $34 and $210 billion a year.

As you can imagine, there is no objective way to measure the severity of depression, as we would do by measuring the frequency of seizures in epilepsy, or the HbA_{1c} levels in diabetes. As an alternative, several questionnaires exist (completed either by the patients or by their physician) that measure the extent of disability associated with depression and the risk for suicide. Although these tools are subjective, many of them provide reasonably accurate measures of depression severity. Unfortunately, these measures are used mainly in the specialist settings. In primary care, where most of depression treatment takes place, formal tools for monitoring depression severity and treatment outcomes are seldom used. More often than not, a crude assessment of whether a change has occurred (I am doing better, I am doing much better, or I am doing worse) is used to determine the success of treatment. However, because depression affects multiple dimensions of a person's life, a more detailed assessment can help focus the treatment for achieving a better outcome.

TREATMENT GOALS

The main desired outcomes in depression are the following:

- Control symptoms
- Improve social and family relationships
- Prevent disability and unemployment
- Prevent suicide

TREATMENT APPROACH

There are several approaches to treating depression, including psychotherapy, pharmacotherapy, and a variety of alternative approaches. A combination of behavioral and pharmacological approaches typically works better than either single approach, but this varies among individuals. Common non–drug treatment approaches such as cognitive behavioral therapy (CBT) and problem-solving therapy can, by themselves, be efficacious. My role here is not to discuss the optimal approach to treating depression or how antidepressants compare in efficacy and safety to nonpharmacological treatments. There are many opinions on the matter. The important point is to recognize that depression is a disorder with potentially serious consequences, and it needs to be treated one way or another. For the purpose of this chapter, I will assume that a decision has been made to pursue antidepressant therapy and will focus on how antidepressant drugs work and how to optimize the pharmacological management of depression.

Antidepressant medications aim to correct the neurotransmitter imbalance in the brain, which is thought to be one of the main mechanisms leading to depression. The key neurotransmitter in this setting is *serotonin*. Serotonin is released from certain neurons in the brain into the space between one neuron and another, which is called a *synapse* (Figure 17.1). By binding to the serotonin receptors located on the neuron on the other side of the synapse, serotonin mediates a certain type of functional "communication" between nerve cells. Usually, serotonin molecules that are not "utilized" are either broken down in the synapse by an enzyme called monoamine oxidase (MAO) or are sucked back (in a process called *reuptake*) to the neuron they were released from, by a protein called the *serotonin transporter*. I am mentioning the terms MAO, *reuptake*, and *serotonin transporter* because they will be required for understanding how the major antidepressant drugs work. Because one of the leading theories in depression suggests an insufficient amount of serotonin in the synapses between brain nerve cells, most treatment approaches are aimed at increasing its amount by utilizing various pharmacological strategies.

Older generations of antidepressants inhibit the enzyme MAO, which breaks down serotonin in the synapse. While this strategy

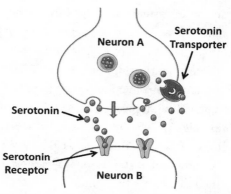

Figure 17.1. A synapse between two neurons. Serotonin in released from neuron A to the synapse and activates serotonin receptors in neuron B. Serotonin transporter mediates the reuptake of extra serotonin back into neuron A. Credit: Elements for this image obtained from Servier image bank: http://www.servier.com/Powerpoint-image-bank.

effectively increases the amount of serotonin, the main problem with MAO inhibitors is that they also inhibit the breakdown of other neuronal transmitters and thus often have additional, potentially serious, side effects. A more successful approach for increasing the effective amount of serotonin in the synapse is by inhibiting the serotonin reuptake back to the neuron. Among the first drugs to do that was *fluoxetine* (Prozac), first approved by the US Food and Drug Administration (FDA) in 1987. The family of drugs that work like *fluoxetine* are called selective serotonin reuptake inhibitors (SSRIs); they block serotonin reuptake to the nerve it was released from, and by doing so, they increase the amount of serotonin in the synapse.

Tricyclic antidepressant (TCA) medications were developed between MAO inhibitors and the SSRI era, mainly in the late 1950s and early 1960s. They have fewer side effects than MAO inhibitors, but their mechanism of action is not as "clean" as that of SSRIs, which means TCAs do inhibit the reuptake of serotonin but affect several other neurotransmitter systems, leading to more side effects. One of those transmitters is acetylcholine, so that many antidepressants cause *anticholinergic* side effects (see Chapter 6) such as dry mouth, constipation, difficulty in urinating, and increased heart rate.

Currently, the initial treatment approach for depression will include taking a single drug, typically an SSRI. This is different from treating, for example, high blood pressure, in which strategies of using lower doses of two or three drugs that work by different mechanisms often prove safer. The reason is that most antidepressant therapies are aimed to increase the content of serotonin. Combining drugs from different antidepressant classes may increase the risk for side effects that these drugs share and potentially the risk for serotonin toxicity, a rare but serious condition called *serotonin syndrome*. Multiple SSRIs exist, but they vary in their characteristics, which can help when adjusting the most appropriate drug to each patient. Table 17.1 summarizes the main available SSRIs as well as some drugs from other groups, such as TCAs and serotonin–norepinephrine reuptake inhibitors (SNRIs), that inhibit the reuptake of not only serotonin, but also norepinephrine, another important neurotransmitter in depression.

SPECIFIC DRUGS
Drug-Related Special Issues

Most antidepressants are long-acting enough to be taken once a day, although in some cases, a twice-daily (or, rarely, 3-times-daily) regimen may be required. As I mentioned, SSRIs somewhat differ in their side-effect profile: some cause sleepiness, and others may cause insomnia. *Fluoxetine* (e.g., Prozac), for example, is among those that may cause restlessness and nervousness. For most people, it would be advisable to take it in the morning to prevent insomnia. *Paroxetine*,

TABLE 17.1 MAIN CATEGORIES OF COMMONLY USED
ANTIDEPRESSANT DRUGS

Drug	Common Doses and Dosing Frequency	Special Instructions and Tips
Selective Serotonin Reuptake Inhibitors (SSRIs)		
Fluoxetine (Prozac, others)	Initiated at 20 mg once a day. Dose may be increased up to 80 mg a day, in one or two daily doses	May cause restlessness, usually taken in the morning
Citalopram (Celexa, others)	20–40 mg, once a day (in patients >60 years old, maximum 20 mg/day is recommended)	
Escitalopram (Lexapro)	10–20 mg once a day	
Paroxetine (Paxil, others)	20 mg, once a day, up to 40–50 mg/day	May cause sleepiness—usually best taken before sleep
Fluvoxamine (Luvox, others)	50–200 mg, in one or two daily doses	Seems to work better in individuals who also have anxiety disorders
Sertraline (Zoloft)	Initiated at 25–50 mg once a day, maintenance at 100–200 mg/day	

(*continued*)

TABLE 17.1 CONTINUED

Drug	Common Doses and Dosing Frequency	Special Instructions and Tips
Serotonin–Norepinephrine Reuptake Inhibitors (SNRIs)		
Venlafaxine (Effexor)	75–375 mg, once or twice a day, depending on formulation*	At higher doses may increase heart rate and blood pressure
Duloxetine (Cymbalta)	60–120 mg, once a day	Might be less effective in smokers (requiring higher doses)
Tricyclic Antidepressants (TCAs)		
Amitriptyline (Elavil, others)	Initiated at 25 mg once a day, maintenance usually at 100–150 mg a day (may be increased in some cases up to 300 mg)	Risk for falls in older adults increases with TCAs. Main side effects: dry mouth, drowsiness, difficulty in urinating, weight gain, constipation. Increased risk for dizziness, especially when standing from lying or sitting position. May increase the risk for seizures and heart rhythm abnormalities (arrhythmias)
Imipramine (Tofranil)	Initiated at 25–75 mg/day, Usual maintenance at 100–150 mg/day. May be increased up to 300 mg/day	
Clomipramine (Anafranil)	Initiated at 25 mg once a day. Usual maintenance at 100–250 mg/day in divided doses to decrease gastrointestinal side effects	

TABLE 17.1 CONTINUED

Drug	Common Doses and Dosing Frequency	Special Instructions and Tips
Desipramine (Norpramin, others)	Initiated at 25–75 mg/day, Usual maintenance at 100–150 mg/day. May be increased up to 300 mg/day	Desipramine and nortriptyline are structurally different from other TCAs in the table. They cause the same types of side effects, but the side effects tend to be milder and less frequent
Nortriptyline (Pamelor)	Initiated at 25–50 mg/day, Usual maintenance at 100-150 mg/day. Higher doses not recommended because potential side effects on the heart	

Commonly Used Other Antidepressants

Drug	Common Doses and Dosing Frequency	Special Instructions and Tips
Bupropion (Wellbutrin, others)	Typically 150–300 mg once a day in slow-release formulation, and 100 mg up to 3 times a day in immediate-release formulation. Maximum 450 mg/day	Affect dopamine and norepinephrine neurotransmitters, with little effect on serotonin. May increase the risk for seizures at high doses

(*continued*)

TABLE 17.1 CONTINUED

Drug	Common Doses and Dosing Frequency	Special Instructions and Tips
Trazodone (Oleptro) and nefazodone (Serzone)	Trazodone: 50 mg 2–3 times a day and can be increased up to 400 mg/day, which can be taken either in two or three doses or once-a-day sustained-release pill. Nefazodone: 100 mg twice a day. Can be increased by 100 mg dose every week to a maximum of 600 mg/day	These drugs usually have minimal *anticholinergic* side effects. Sleepiness and dizziness (with blood pressure decrease) when standing from lying or sitting are the most common side effects. Rarely may cause liver damage and *priapism* (involuntary, painful erection)
Mirtazapine (Remeron)	Started at 15 mg once a day before bedtime, can be increased up to 45 mg/day. Older adults (especially men) and individuals with kidney problems should get reduced doses	Mechanism of action differs from other antidepressants. Directly activates some serotonin receptors but affects other neurotransmitters such as norepinephrine as well. Somnolence is the most common side effect. Also may cause weight gain, dry mouth, and constipation

on the other hand, is typically more sedating. It would be less recommended in the morning and therefore is often taken in the evening to avoid daytime sleepiness. In addition, individuals with mixed anxiety and depression may benefit more from paroxetine because of its sedating effect.

It is also important to recognize that some SSRIs are prone to more drug–drug interactions than others. This is particularly true for *fluvoxamine, fluoxetine,* and *paroxetine.* These are metabolized by CYP enzymes, and drugs that can inhibit or induce CYP enzymes (see Chapter 8) can change SSRI blood concentrations and thus effectiveness. In addition, these SSRIs are themselves strong inhibitors of CYP enzymes and can impair the metabolism of other drugs. Therefore, if you are taking other medications, consult your doctor on the optimal choice of your antidepressant to avoid unnecessary drug–drug interactions.

Some antidepressants may cause nervousness in the first days, or even weeks, of treatment. It is not uncommon to see doctors prescribe a sedative or antianxiety drug (benzodiazepines, e.g., *clonazepam*) for this initial period. It is important to understand that the objective of this additional treatment is to mitigate the side effects associated with new SSRI therapy. Therefore, these benzodiazepines should be used at low doses and for a limited period of time.

MAO inhibitor antidepressants are not routinely used and are typically reserved for the most difficult, treatment-resistant cases. MAO inhibitors are associated with many safety issues, including (1) a very long action (weeks), which does not allow much room for adjustments if therapy needs to be discontinued; (2) multiple drug–drug interactions; and (3) interaction with certain types of food and beverages, such as wine and cheeses, which can lead to very high blood pressure.

TCAs (e.g., *amitriptyline, clomipramine, desipramine, imipramine*) had been the most commonly used drugs before the late 1980s. They have a mixed profile of action mechanisms and are often quite effective at appropriate doses. However, TCAs have the potential for multiple side effects, including dry mouth, weight gain, decrease in libido, sleepiness, dizziness, heart rate problems at higher doses, constipation, difficulty in urinating, and other effects. Despite the abundance of potential side effects, people often tolerate many of these side effects if TCAs are initiated at low doses, and their dose is slowly increased over a period of several weeks. Starting TCA therapy at high doses almost inevitably leads to stopping the treatment because of side effects.

With the appearance of the first SSRI on the market, the treatment of depression has shifted gears. The SSRIs are usually much better tolerated than the older generation of antidepressants; they do not cause as many side effects and have less varied dosing regimens. SSRIs are currently recommended as first-line treatment for depression, together with a similar group of drugs called SNRIs (e.g., *duloxetine* and *venlafaxine*).

In people in whom SSRIs or SNRIs fail to reasonably control the symptoms of depression, the strategy can include switching to another SSRI or an SNRI. If one SSRI does not work, that does not mean that another won't. Alternatively, other medications from Table 17.1 are considered, either by switching to another single drug or by combining an SSRI with another medication, such as *bupropion, mirtazapine,* or *trazodone*. It may be safer to combine a drug that works on serotonin (e.g., SSRI) with a drug that works on a different neurotransmitter to prevent too much serotonergic stimulation.

As I mentioned earlier in this chapter, drug treatment for depression will usually be initiated with a single antidepressant. An important point related to the effectiveness of antidepressant drugs is that it may take up to 6 weeks to begin experiencing improvement from the treatment. As you can imagine, quite a lot of patience is required to see whether one drug works. The same is true if someone switches from one antidepressant to another. It may take several weeks to titrate the drug to reach a reasonable and tolerable dose, and a few more weeks until the full extent of clinical effect is achieved. This is a critical point because some people will try a new medication and stop it if they don't experience significant relief of their depression symptoms within 1 or 2 weeks.

Potential Safety Issues

Serotonin, in addition to its effect in the brain, also has a role in blood clotting. Platelets in the blood require serotonin to aggregate and form blood clots. SSRIs may block the entry of serotonin to the platelet and thus impair appropriate blood clotting. Since *aspirin*, nonsteroidal anti-inflammatory drugs (NSAIDs), and additional drugs such as *clopidogrel* (Plavix) also prevent platelet aggregation, the combination may increase the risk for bleeding, especially stomach bleeds (see Chapter 13). If you are treated with an antidepressant drug and are now prescribed aspirin or an NSAID, ask your provider about your risk for bleeding.

TCAs and SSRIs may negatively affect libido and erectile function and can cause difficulties in ejaculation. If undesired effects occur, often a change in dose or a switch to another antidepressant under your doctor's supervision can be beneficial.

Although it is a quite rare event, if you are treated with antidepressants, you should be aware of *serotonin syndrome*. It usually occurs when an antidepressant has been combined with another serotonergic drug, either another antidepressant or other drug that affects serotonin (e.g., *tramadol* for treating pain, or certain types of antibiotics like *linezolid*). The syndrome can progress quite rapidly. It usually includes hyperthermia (increase in body temperature), increase in blood pressure, muscle stiffness or twitching, changes in blood pressure, and mental status changes, such as nervousness and confusion. If these symptoms and signs are suspected, immediate medical intervention is required—call 911.

During my work in intensive care unit, I have encountered only two such cases, and both included the intake of two long-acting antidepressants. Unfortunately, both cases were life-threatening and required intubation (connection to artificial ventilation) and sedation for several days in the intensive care until the patients were stabilized. There are currently no tools to identify high-risk individuals who are more likely to develop serotonin syndrome; thousands of patients could receive the same combination of antidepressants, but only a few would develop this severe condition. Therefore, the general approach should be the attempt to avoid multiple serotonergic medications (to the extent possible) and to increase patient awareness to seek medical care if symptoms are noticed.

SPECIAL POPULATIONS

Women with Postpartum Depression

Depression after delivering a baby is a quite common phenomenon and may require antidepressant treatment. SSRIs are usually the drugs of choice. If the decision, on consulting with your doctor, is that you will need antidepressant treatment, in most of cases you will be able to continue breastfeeding (if you choose to) because the amount of the drug that reaches the breast milk is quite low and is not associated with negative consequences in the breastfeeding baby. *Paroxetine* and *sertraline* seem to be associated with very low or undetectable drug levels in the breastfeeding infant's blood and might be advisable, pending no contraindications or other considerations that would require alternative treatment.

Adolescents

Escitalopram and *fluoxetine* are approved for treating depression in adolescents. The FDA has issued a special warning that treatment with SSRIs may increase the risk for suicidal thoughts and suicide in adolescents, especially in the first 4 weeks of treatment. Therefore, closer monitoring on behalf of parents and caregivers is required during the first month of therapy. In general, SSRIs are well tolerated by adolescents.

Older Adults

Older adult patients are more likely to experience drug side effects in general. If a drug causes drowsiness, older adult patients are more likely to fall, which can result in serious injuries. Anticholinergic side effects such as constipation and difficulty in urinating are also more common and profound in older adults. SSRIs are usually preferable to TCAs in older adults because of fewer sedating effects. On the other hand, SSRIs are sometimes associated with drop in blood sodium levels (hyponatremia), and older adult patients are at a higher risk for this effect, so monitoring of symptoms such as confusion, muscle weakness, or tremor (shaking) might be necessary. If a TCA is indicated in an older adult patient, it will be usually initiated at low doses (one half to one fourth of the regular adult dose). Treatment should be monitored carefully, mainly for increased risks for falls and heart rhythm abnormalities.

Patients with Treatment-Resistant Depression

Some patients may try several types of antidepressants, as well as a combination of psychotherapy and pharmacotherapy, and still not improve. Patients who do not improve after a full-dose trial of two or more antidepressants are usually considered as suffering from *treatment-resistant depression.* Additional approaches exist to "augment" the antidepressant management in these patients. I will not discuss them in length, but only mention that your psychiatrist might consider using drugs from other classes that have been shown to help improve the therapeutic effect of antidepressants. These augmentation therapies have been used with a variable degree of success and include drugs such as *lithium* (mainly used for bipolar disorder), *thyroid hormones* (see Chapter 19), *valproate* or *carbamazepine* (antiepileptic drugs; see Chapter 16), and *olanzapine.*

The tipping point of balance between improvement of symptoms and prevention of suicidal thoughts, and between potential side effects from the additional treatment, is going to be determined based on your individual conditions and preferences. When additional medications are considered for treatment-resistant depression, many people may feel that this is a vicious circle of adding more medications, which may add more side effects, which will then require even more medications to treat the side effects. It is therefore very important to consult with experienced physicians and consider exploring possible nonpharmacological treatment options as well.

IMPORTANT QUESTIONS TO ASK YOUR DOCTOR

- What are the milestones for determining that my treatment is successful?
- What changes can I make in my daily routine to help my antidepressant treatment be more successful?
- Are there medications I need to avoid because of my current treatment?

- Are there periodic tests I should undergo to ensure safety of my antidepressant drug(s)?

THINGS YOU CAN DO TO IMPROVE TREATMENT OUTCOMES

As with many other conditions, it is important to monitor treatment outcomes. Research shows that quite often, depression symptoms are not monitored with appropriate tools. Because several social, emotional, and physical aspects are affected by depression, it is important to determine whether the treatment goals are achieved on each of these dimensions. There are a variety of validated tools that can help your doctor better assess the changes in your depression over time. These are typically questionnaires that you fill out as accurately as possible, and they provide valuable information on your symptoms, resulting in a score that can be tracked over time. A variety of such questionnaires exist, including the Hamilton Depression Rating Scale, the Beck Depression Inventory, and others. Because no lab test or brain imaging test can provide objective information on your depression symptoms and severity, routine use of one of these questionnaires can provide a valuable tool in fine-tuning your treatment to maximize its success.

If the goals are not achieved, it might be worth considering alternative or additional (pharmacological or nonpharmacological) treatments to better control your symptoms and improve your quality of life.

There are also changes in lifestyle that can help your treatment success. Although depression negatively affects peoples' desire to be physically active, studies consistently show that routine exercise (even moderate activity such as walking) improves depression symptoms. Incorporating exercise in your daily routine can substantially help improve your symptoms in the long run.

The effectiveness of some antidepressant drugs such as *duloxetine* may be decreased in smokers because chronic smoking causes an induction of certain CYP enzymes in the liver. Therefore, smokers may not achieve full benefit of the treatment or may need higher doses than nonsmokers for obtaining an appropriate antidepressant effect.

VALUABLE RESOURCES FOR ADDITIONAL EDUCATION ON DEPRESSION

National Institute of Mental Health: https://www.nimh.nih.gov/ health/topics/depression/index.shtml

A wonderful free booklet on depression: https://www.nimh.nih. gov/health/publications/depression-what-you-need-to-know/ index.shtml

National Alliance on Mental Illness: http://www.nami.org/Learn-More/Mental-Health-Conditions/Depression

[18]

DOES IT REALLY HAVE
TO HURT?

Managing Pain Wisely

Almost everyone experiences pain from time to time whether from an accidental injury, headache, or sore back. In fact, about 90% of the adult population experience at least one episode of acute pain a month. Unlike many other of the disorders we've discussed so far, *pain* has a critical evolutionary function that is necessary for survival: to warn us about tissue damage or inflammatory processes. Despite the importance of recognizing its biological role, pain is an unpleasant sensory and emotional experience, and the suffering caused by it is mostly unnecessary. For example, chest pain is a warning sign for a heart attack. If you come to the emergency department with chest pain and a suspected heart attack, there is no benefit to continue suffering from pain. In fact, one of the first treatments you would get at that point is intravenous *morphine* to relieve the chest pain. And it's not only the unpleasant experience that will be improved: untreated pain causes a variety of negative outcomes, such as anxiety, elevation in blood pressure, increase in heart rate, and difficulty in taking deep breaths. Treating pain timely and effectively can prevent negative consequences beyond merely relieving the suffering. I will first briefly discuss interventions for managing acute pain, but the main focus of this chapter is on the treatment of chronic pain.

ACUTE PAIN

Acute pain outside the hospital is often treated with over-the counter (OTC) medications. Among the painkillers most commonly used for acute (or short-term) pain are *acetaminophen* (Tylenol, others), and nonsteroidal anti-inflammatory drugs (NSAIDs) such as *ibuprofen* (Advil, Motrin, others) and *naproxen* (Aleve, others). NSAIDs are the most frequently used drugs in the world, highlighting on one hand how common pain is, and on the other hand how unpleasant it is, so that people frequently take mediations to relieve it. As outlined in Chapter 9, you should take all the appropriate precautions when using OTC medications as you would with a prescription medication. While OTC painkillers are usually safe when taken in recommended doses for a short period of time, there are some potential risks you should be aware of. I will briefly describe how these medications work to help illustrate their undesired effects as well.

First, *acetaminophen* (also called *paracetamol*) is quite different from the other analgesics such as *ibuprofen* or *naproxen*, which are NSAIDs. While you should not combine two different NSAIDs on the same day (because they share side effects and your risk for side effects will increase), acetaminophen has a different side-effect profile, and in some cases your physician or pharmacist can recommend combining acetaminophen with an NSAID, if the pain is not relieved by either of the drugs alone.

NSAIDs reduce pain and inflammation by inhibiting an enzyme called cyclooxygenase (COX), which is responsible for producing major inflammatory molecules in the body. COX is associated with inflammation but also has important physiological functions in the body related to kidney function, stomach protection from acid, and blood clotting. The inhibition of the COX enzyme by NSAIDs, especially with long-term or high-dose treatment, can damage the protective lining in our stomach and the upper intestine and increase the risk for stomach ulcers or bleeding. In addition, COX inhibition may prolong bleeding in general, and impair kidney function. Importantly, it has been discovered that there are two types of COX enzymes: one of them, COX-1 is mainly involved in the physiological (protective) activity, and the other one, COX-2, is mainly involved in mediating pain and inflammation. Unfortunately, most NSAIDs inhibit both forms of COX, resulting in reduction of both pain and inflammation, but also in side effects.

Because COX enzyme is involved in blood clotting and stomach protection, NSAIDs are particularly risky and may cause stomach or intestinal bleeding in patients with preexisting stomach ulcers, especially patients who receive blood thinners such as aspirin and antidepressants such as SSRIs (see Chapter 17). It is estimated that between 70,000 and 100,000 hospitalizations a year occur in the United States due to gastrointestinal complications of NSAIDs, 7600 to 15,000 of which result in patient death. Newer data from the United Kingdom indicate that in younger patients these numbers may have improved over the past 10 years, perhaps owing to more awareness, but in older adults, the risks for NSAID-associated stomach bleeding are still high. Additionally, long-term use of NSAIDs is associated with potential kidney damage and mildly increased risk for heart attack and stroke.

A newer class of prescription-only analgesics, COX-2 selective inhibitors such as *celecoxib* (Celebrex) or *etoricoxib* (Arcoxia, available in Europe), pose a lower risk for stomach ulcers and bleeding. However, other risks, such as kidney damage and heart attack, may not be different between selective COX-2 inhibitors and traditional, nonselective COX inhibitors (NSAIDs). If you have gastrointestinal problems such as stomach ulcers (or even had them in the past), you should not use NSAIDs without consulting your physician. If you need an analgesic or anti-inflammatory treatment, your physician might consider prescribing a COX-2 inhibitor for you and potentially add a stomach-protecting drug such as *omeprazole* (Prilosec, others) or *lansoprazole* (Prevacid, others) to reduce the risk for gastrointestinal bleeding.

In certain conditions in which the injured tissue is close to the skin surface, for example, a muscle strain or knee pain, NSAID creams or gels such as *diclofenac* (Voltaren) can be applied to the painful area to achieve somewhat similar pain relief, but without the undesired effects on the stomach, the kidney, or blood clotting. The topical cream can help achieving a similar local anti-inflammatory effect in the injured area, while minimizing drug exposure to other organs. With application of recommended cream doses to the skin, a similar drug concentration in the muscle or knee joint can be achieved, but with 80 to 90% less systemic exposure.

Acetaminophen, on the other hand, is not an NSAID. It does not reduce inflammation, and it relieves pain by a somewhat different mechanism than NSAIDs. Acetaminophen also reduces fever, as NSAIDs do. The side-effect profile of acetaminophen is also quite different from NSAIDs. It is a very safe drug in doses below 4 g/day and does not have the gastrointestinal and heart risks that are associated with NSAIDs. However, doses higher than recommended may cause liver damage, especially if you already have an existing liver problem such as hepatitis. *Acetaminophen* overdose may result in fatal liver damage, if not treated in a timely manner.

If you have an acute pain condition for which a treatment with *acetaminophen* or NSAIDs is not efficacious enough or is not possible because of other conditions and medications, your doctor may prescribe other types of medications to relieve your pain. These may be muscle relaxants, if the pain is due to stiff muscles, or medications such as *opioids*, which are discussed more thoroughly in the chronic pain section.

CHRONIC PAIN

Unlike acute pain, which can be reasonably managed in most situations, long-lasting **chronic pain** is much more challenging. It is not currently known whether there is any physiological "value" (or gain) in chronic pain, or rather if it is a result of maladaptive responses of our nervous system to the initial injury that triggered the pain. Many times, the initial tissue injury has healed, but the person continues to suffer from long-term pain. Interestingly, two people may have apparently the same extent of tissue damage (e.g., the same appearance of a knee radiograph in arthritis), but one person will experience long-term pain and the other will not. We do not currently understand the exact biological processes responsible for these individual differences, but it is quite clear that the injury itself is not the only contributor. There are a variety of genetic, psychological, and social factors that contribute to the development of chronic pain. These factors need to be addressed in chronic pain management programs, although treatment approaches addressing these are beyond the scope of this book.

Chronic pain is very common; large surveys demonstrate that 20 to 25% of adults worldwide suffer from chronic pain at any given point in time. Given that chronic pain costs the US economy more than $500 billion annually, it can justify the "biggest health problem" label quite effortlessly.

Among the most common chronic pain conditions are headaches (including migraine headaches); musculoskeletal conditions such as back, neck, and joint pain; and various types of pain due to nerve damage (called *neuropathic* pain). An additional group of chronic pain conditions includes somewhat less well-defined but common syndromes such as *fibromyalgia, irritable bowel syndrome,* and *chronic pelvic pain.* As you can see, chronic pain can be caused by a variety of pathologies. It is not surprising, therefore, that approaches to treating each chronic pain syndrome are unique. Although this chapter cannot review the various subtypes of pain and their treatment guidelines, there are some nuances that are important to understand for improving the safety and the outcomes of chronic pain management. I will focus on these. You will find that *neuropathic* pain has received more attention in this chapter, and the reason is that while in many types of pain nonpharmacological interventions have an increasingly important role, in *neuropathic* pain the current evidence suggests that drug therapy remains the key approach.

TREATMENT GOALS

When initiating **any** analgesic therapy for **chronic pain**, it is critical to determine how much your **functional level** and **quality of life** change following the treatment. Medications for chronic pain are often not treating the underlying condition but are providing symptom relief. This relief can be important in allowing you to perform physical therapy or other rehabilitation activity but should be treated as such. Every new drug should start as a trial, and its benefits versus side effects need to be carefully assessed. If after a few weeks of maintenance on the target dose, the daily use of a drug results in substantial pain relief and objective improvement in functioning, it is then worth considering long-term treatment with the drug. If no such positive effect is achieved or the improvement is only minimal with no functional benefits, it is *strongly advised* to talk to your doctor and discuss discontinuing the treatment. The exception is when your doctor decides to try a combination of treatments and, in case of partial relief with one drug, adds a trial of a second (or third) drug with a different mechanism to complement the treatment. But even if this is the case, you must carefully monitor how much improvement the drugs provide and continue the treatment only when a clear benefit exists. You, as the patient suffering from the pain, are the *only* person who can determine how beneficial an intervention is. It is easy (and common) to get used to taking drugs that have only mild effects. Many people take analgesics for years and don't even know how their pain feels without the drug. Some of those who attempt gradual discontinuation are surprised to discover that their pain is the same or even better without the pain medications; plus, stopping the drugs provides the bonus of eliminating their side effects.

I will repeat my mantra: *if you cannot measure it, you cannot improve it.* Pain, like depression, cannot be assessed by objective tools; unfortunately, there is no *pain-o-meter.* Therefore, it is important to determine how much the pain interferes with various aspects of your life and to set individual goals of what would be a desirable treatment outcome. Setting meaningful expectations is also important. Just as patients cannot expect that their diabetes or high blood pressure will simply disappear with treatment, it is also often the case with chronic pain. Setting a realistic goal of controlling (instead of eliminating) pain to achieve a reasonable level of functioning can actually help the recovery process. Patients, who have suffered with pain for years, often expect their new or next treatment to completely resolve their pain. More often than not, such high expectations result in frustration and increased anxiety. If the new treatment reduces the pain intensity by half, one can be left very satisfied or very disappointed with the outcome, depending on the initial expectations. My best advice would be to set up realistic goals for each treatment phase and do your best to achieve these, one goal at a time.

TREATMENT APPROACH

Based on the diagnosis of your painful condition, the treatment approach will vary. Physical therapy and exercise may offer substantial help in many chronic pain syndromes. Long-term pain is often associated with behavioral and even cognitive changes; therefore, behavioral assessment, improvement in coping skills, and cognitive-behavioral treatments are all beneficial. Also, complementary approaches such as (but not limited to) acupuncture, tai chi, massage therapy, and biofeedback have shown effectiveness in different chronic pain settings. There are interventional approaches such as epidural injections for low back and leg pain, radiofrequency ablation of inflamed nerves, or spinal cord stimulation for various diagnoses, but these are beyond the focus of this chapter. This chapter will focus on improving the effectiveness and the safety of medications for managing chronic pain.

Pain from Muscles, Bones, and Joints (Musculoskeletal Pain)

When you suffer from pain of musculoskeletal origin (perhaps with the exception of cancer-related pain), relying exclusively on analgesic drugs for long-term control of your pain is quite a *bad* idea. Research clearly shows that pain medications alone are not going to improve your condition much over time. Instead, analgesic medications should be used to reduce pain sufficiently to allow for physical therapy, exercise, and rehabilitation activities. This is conceptually difficult to accept because this approach will require very active involvement and responsibility on your behalf. And this is where many patients are trapped. Some patients may not have enough resources, motivation, or time (you name it) to be actively involved in treatment programs aimed to improve their long-term outcomes, and instead only rely on analgesics, often in increasing doses, to control their pain. Unfortunately, prescribers often have limited ability to offer rehabilitative or multidisciplinary approaches to pain and hence tend to prescribe more analgesics when initial treatment is not working. In my opinion, this is one of the main reasons behind the current epidemic of opioid analgesic–related overdoses and deaths in the Western world. As I mentioned earlier, each analgesic drug should be initiated as a trial, with clear goals of **functional** improvement. No substantial improvement means no chronic treatment with the drug.

I will discuss the following groups of medications for the treatment of chronic musculoskeletal pain: *NSAIDs, acetaminophen, muscle relaxants,* and *opioids* (with the latter meriting the most detailed description).

Nonopioid Medications
NSAIDs can be very helpful to reduce the pain enough to allow physical activity and rehabilitation exercises. A variety of OTC and prescription NSAIDs (e.g., *diclofenac, etodolac, meloxicam, nabumetone*) are available. However, the long-term use of these drugs increases the risk for stomach ulcers and bleeding, and *COX-2 enzyme inhibitors* such as *celecoxib* may be a safer alternative. Because prolonged use of high-dose NSAIDs may also be associated with an increased risk for kidney damage, heart attack, and stroke, it is usually advised to limit the use of NSAIDs (or COX-2 inhibitors) for short periods of time and not to take them daily for long periods.

Acetaminophen (paracetamol) usually provides mild to moderate pain relief but does not reduce inflammation, as opposed to NSAIDs. On the other hand, *acetaminophen* is much safer with long-term use than NSAIDs and is a good alternative if it provides sufficient enough pain relief for your condition. The main issue with *acetaminophen* is the importance of paying attention to the daily dose you use. Although very safe at regular doses, using more than 4 g/day in adults increases the risk for liver damage. Children require special attention as well because the maximum daily dose is determined by the child's weight. It is also important to remember that acetaminophen is included in many combination drugs both for pain and for cold and flu. You should make sure the *total acetaminophen* dose does not exceed 4 g/day for an adult.

Muscle relaxants are commonly used in the acute pain setting, particularly for low back pain, but very little evidence exists to support their long-term benefits in chronic pain. Muscle relaxants are actually indicated for short-term management of acute pain (for 1 to 3 weeks) but in fact are more commonly prescribed long-term for chronic pain. Many muscle relaxants cause drowsiness, especially when combined with other sedatives and alcohol. In addition, their long-term use may result in physical and psychological dependence. There is really no good evidence to suggest that one muscle relaxant is better than another. The commonly used ones are *carisoprodol* (Soma), *methocarbamol* (Robaxan), *orphenadrine* (Norflex, Norgesic), *cyclobenzapril, baclofen, diazepam,* and *tizanidine* (Zanaflex), and some are available in combination with NSAIDs or *codeine*. When acute pain is associated with muscle tightness or spasms, these drugs can be useful, but the evidence to suggest their benefit with chronic use is questionable. You should thoroughly discuss the benefits versus risks of muscle relaxants with your physician, if these drugs are to be prescribed for your chronic pain.

Opioid Medications

Opioids, with *morphine* being the representative drug of the group, are the strongest painkillers known to humankind. One exception would be general anesthesia, which essentially turns your consciousness off.

Initially isolated from the *opium* poppy (hence the name), today a variety of natural and synthetic opioids exist for managing pain. Opioids are often used for acute pain such as trauma, chest pain during a heart attack, or pain after surgery. They are also quite common in treating cancer-related moderate to severe pain. However, in some cases, opioids can be useful in treating chronic pain that is not related to cancer. Opioids were infrequently prescribed for this kind of pain before the 1990s, but around that time it was recognized that chronic pain is quite undertreated globally, and among the efforts to improve the management of pain, there has been a push to prescribe opioids more aggressively, and some would argue—recklessly. As I described in Chapter 6, opioids may cause serious side effects, including addiction and death. As the wide use of opioids increased, prescription opioid-related deaths rose sharply in the past two decades in the United States, Canada, United Kingdom, and other countries in what has been termed the *opioid epidemic*. The National Action Plan for Adverse Drug Event Prevention (ADE Action Plan) has identified opioids as one of the three most significant areas of patient safety concern with medications. To illustrate the significance of this point, the number of deaths from *prescription* opioid analgesics in the United Stated has **quadrupled** in about a decade and a half, from around 4000 deaths a year in 1999 to more than 16,000 deaths in 2015. Below, I outline some of the opioid risks to help you make informed decisions and keep away from these horrifying statistics (Table 18.1 describes the most common opioid analgesics available).

Opioids are controlled substances, which means that they can cause physical and psychological dependence, especially when used long-term. This is not to say they should not be prescribed, but it does mean that the risks should be carefully weighed against benefits for each individual. Here is my advice on 10 key issues to consider for improving the safety of opioid treatment for chronic pain:

TABLE 18.1 COMMON TYPES OF OPIOID ANALGESICS

Type of Opioid	Examples	Comments
Strong opioid (oral)	Morphine, oxycodone (OxyContin), hydromorphone (Dilaudid), methadone, oxymorphone (Opana)	Comes in a variety of long-acting and short-acting formulations. Methadone side effects need to be monitored even more carefully for the first weeks after initiating treatment and at each dose increase
Strong opioid + acetaminophen (oral)	Oxycodone with acetaminophen (Percocet), hydrocodone + acetaminophen (Vicodin)	Short-acting. Provides pain relief for 3 to 6 hours. Pay attention to total daily acetaminophen dose (from any product) not to exceed 4 grams
Strong opioid (skin patch)	Fentanyl (Durogesic) Buprenorphine (Butrans)	Fentanyl patches need to be replaced every 72 hours (3 days) Buprenorphine patches need to be replaced every 7 days. Apply the patch on a relatively nonhairy skin (upper back, shoulder, upper chest), and rotate the location of each new patch. It takes 8–12 hours from first (or new dose) patch placement to feel the full effect. The drug released under the skin is active for 8–12 hours after patch removal

TABLE 18.1 CONTINUED

Type of Opioid	Examples	Comments
Weak opioid	Tramadol	Prescribed for moderate to severe pain. Tramadol does have a maximum dose—up to 400 mg/day. Drug interactions occur with a variety of drugs, including antidepressants
	Codeine	Use for pain is currently discouraged. Weak analgesic. Unpredictable effect

1. You must **start low and go slow** in terms of opioid dose. Even if you are in a lot of pain, NEVER take doses higher (or more frequently) than you have been prescribed, and NEVER increase the daily dose faster than recommended by your physician. Your body may gradually get used to some opioid side effects, but **gradually** is the key word.

2. Too high of an opioid dose may cause you to **stop breathing;** this is what usually causes opioid-related deaths. Opioids interfere with the function of the respiration control center in the brainstem. This phenomenon of **respiratory depression** will typically not occur if you are treated with the same dose of opioid for a long time and if nothing has changed in terms of your medical condition or other drugs you take. It is usually a consequence of starting with too high of a dose (either for the first time or after not taking opioids for a while), increasing the dose too fast, having a medical condition that affects breathing or impairs kidney or liver function, or

experiencing drug interactions that increase the concentration or the respiratory effect of the opioid. The **respiratory depression** from opioids typically occurs while a person is asleep at night or feels tired and drowsy and becomes sleepy and unresponsive. If another person lives at home with an opioid-treated individual, it is very important to educate this person about respiratory depression. Healthy adults take around 12 to 16 breaths a minute. There is some variability, but if an opioid-treated individual's respiratory rate is *less than 8 breaths per minute,* this is considered an emergency, and an attempt must be made to wake the person. If the individual is nonresponsive at this point, call emergency services immediately. If an opioid-treated person becomes drowsy and nonresponsive to stimuli such as calling by name, shaking, or pinching, the person must be rushed to a hospital (or call 911), even if the breathing rate is higher than 8 breaths a minute. Emergency services will stabilize the patient and administer the opioid antagonist *naloxone* to treat the overdose. It is important to know that *naloxone* is also available in a self-administered injection (Evzio), which can be self-injected or injected by another person in the case of suspected opioid overdose. In several countries and US states, an OTC naloxone nasal spray is also available for the emergency treatment of an opioid overdose. It may be a good idea to discuss a *naloxone* prescription with your doctor if you are treated with opioids, especially at high doses.

3. There is no formal maximum dose for most opioids because there are **huge differences among individuals** in terms of response to opioids. Although prescriptions for high doses of opioids are tightly regulated to prevent overdose, the doses are personalized to each individual. One person may have severe side effects from 20 mg/day of *oxycodone,* while another

may have minimal side effects from 100 mg/day of *oxycodone* (provided the dose was achieved by slow titration). Many factors contribute to these individual differences, including genetics, age, weight, prior exposure to opioids, existing medical conditions, and the use of other drugs. Therefore, it is critical that you don't use an opioid analgesic that was prescribed to another person and don't share your opioids with someone else. A dose that is safe for you may be fatal for another person, and vice versa. Keep your opioids in a safe location that is not accessible to occasional visitors to your home.

4. Despite the previously mentioned risks, lawfully prescribed and **appropriately monitored** opioid treatment can often be safe. But there is a justification for taking opioids long-term, ONLY when there is a clear functional improvement associated with substantial relief of pain and no or minimal side effects. A clear plan for frequent and appropriate assessment of side effects, as well as of the functional improvement with the treatment, is the key to safe opioid use for chronic pain. Please remember: opioid therapy for chronic pain is not a life sentence without a possibility of parole. If the treatment does not work safely, or the pain relief is only marginal, opioids can (and should) be discontinued.

5. **Constipation.** Most people who are treated with opioids for more than a few days will develop constipation. Therefore, it is a good idea to start with constipation prevention in parallel with opioids. Products based on *senna, bisacodyl* (Dulcolax, others), *polyethylene glycol* (PEG, MiraLAX), or *lactulose* (Constulose, others) usually work well. There are opioid products (e.g., Targin, Targiniq) that are strong analgesics and include an inherent compound that blocks the opioid effects on the gut to reduce constipation.

6. **Androgen deficiency**. Long-term opioid treatment often causes a decrease in male and female sex hormone (e.g., testosterone, luteinizing hormone) levels, causing tiredness, reduction in sexual drive (libido), or erectile dysfunction in men. It is important to diagnose this condition because it can be potentially managed by switching to another opioid, reducing opioid doses, or administering hormone replacement therapy.

7. **Understand dependence, tolerance, and addiction**. These effects are among the biggest concerns with opioid treatment. I would like to make some clarifications, at least in the terminology. *Dependence* is a natural (physiologic) phenomenon that occurs with many drugs. It means that if you suddenly stop using the drug, you will experience side effects of a *withdrawal* reaction. This reaction happens with steroid drugs, some medications to treat hypertension, and others. Dependence per se does not mean addiction.

   Tolerance is a different beast. It usually means that the individual needs increasing doses of the drug to achieve the same effect. There are several explanations as to why this happens, but for most drugs, there is no solution for this phenomenon. It is important to differentiate between the worsening of a patient's pain and the development of tolerance because both will eventually require an increase in opioid dose. If you develop tolerance to your opioids treatment (and need increasing doses to control pain), it is usually not a good sign for long-term benefit from opioid treatment and puts you at a higher risk for serious side effects. It may also mean that opioids may be making your pain worse (a term called *opioid-induced hyperalgesia*). If that happens, you should discuss nonopioid treatment options with your doctor and approaches to taper-off your opioids.

Addiction is quite a distinct concept that implies continued use of a drug despite ongoing harm caused by it. Addiction typically has psychological and behavioral characteristics as well, such as craving when a dose was missed, drug seeking, taking higher doses than prescribed, and using illegal methods to obtain the drug or prescriptions. Addiction is a serious condition that should be addressed and treated as soon as possible.

8. **Don't discontinue opioids abruptly**. After you have been treated for a few weeks or longer, opioids should be tapered down gradually. Your doctor will instruct you based on your individual circumstances, but as a rule of thumb, reducing about 20% (one fifth) of the daily dose every 7 to 10 days can be a reasonable starting point. For example, if you take 100 mg of drug X, your doctor may guide you to reduce the dose to 80 mg a day for a week, then 65 mg a day for another week, 50 mg a day for a week, and so on. You may find out that you need to stay on each dose level for 2 to 3 weeks (or longer) to avoid side effects, and ask your physician for an even slower taper. Abrupt discontinuation may cause the pain to get worse, increase heart rate and blood pressure, and cause nervousness, difficulty sleeping and concentrating, cold sweats, diarrhea, and other symptoms.

9. **Be attentive to the amount of acetaminophen in combination doses**. Several opioid drugs (Vicodin, Percocet) contain acetaminophen (paracetamol). Depending on the number of tablets you take in a day, acetaminophen can reach substantial amounts. If you are taking prescription or OTC acetaminophen, make sure that the total daily dose does not exceed 4000 mg (4 grams).

10. **Avoid alcohol and minimize sedative drugs**. The risk for respiratory depression from opioids substantially increases with alcohol and different sedative drugs such as benzodiazepines like *diazepam* (Valium), *clonazepam* (Klonopin), and others, or muscle relaxants. The combination with alcohol or sedatives also impairs alertness and concentration to a significant degree.

Neuropathic Pain

Musculoskeletal pain typically results from inflammatory processes affecting the muscles, bones, and joints, causing the nerve cells (neurons) to transmit the information about that injury to the brain. Neuropathic pain, on the other hand, results from direct damage to the nerves due to a disease or trauma. The damaged nerve cells (neurons) generate the "painful" electrical signals that travel to the brain to create the pain experience. Among leading neuropathic pain conditions are *painful neuropathies* causing pain in the feet (and sometimes the hands), in what is called a "stocking-glove" distribution. This "symmetric" nerve damage may result from a variety of causes, such as diabetes, HIV/AIDS, alcoholism, or certain anticancer drugs. Additional common causes for neuropathic pain are shingles (zoster) infection, spinal cord injury, stroke, and nerve damage due to trauma or surgery.

Neuropathic pain often feels different from inflammatory pain; it is commonly described as electric shock–like, burning, stabbing, numb, or like *pins and needles*. Your doctor may perform some tests on your skin or send you for a nerve conduction study to confirm the diagnosis of neuropathic pain. The drugs used for treating neuropathic pain are usually not the analgesics like NSAIDs or *acetaminophen* that we described earlier. The two main groups of drugs for treating neuropathic pain are antidepressants (see Chapter 17) and antiepileptic drugs (see Chapter 16). The rationale for the use of these drug categories in neuropathic pain is the following:

1. In the damaged nervous system, the neurons that usually respond to painful stimuli, become hyperactive, and generate electrical impulses on their own. This is somewhat similar to what happens in epilepsy, but the hyperactive neurons in epilepsy are responsible for muscle function, and the hyperactive neurons in neuropathic pain are responsible for transmitting painful sensations. Since most antiepileptic drugs reduce the activity of hyperactive nerve cells in general, many of them can also help in neuropathic pain.

2. The nerve damage and the ongoing neuropathic pain result in imbalance of several neural messengers (neurotransmitters), such as norepinephrine and serotonin in the brain and the spinal cord. Certain antidepressant drugs can help restore this imbalance, although not all antidepressants are effective for neuropathic pain. The selective serotonin reuptake inhibitor (SSRI) antidepressants (see Chapter 17) don't seem to help, but the serotonin–norepinephrine reuptake inhibitor (SNRI) antidepressants and tricyclic antidepressants (TCAs) are efficacious and are described in Table 18.2. The table describes the most recommended ones and some of the important issues regarding their use for pain.

Opioids can be used for treating neuropathic pain, but they are usually not the treatment of choice because of the safety concerns described previously.

In general, neuropathic pain is challenging to treat. The process of identifying the effective drug (or drug combination) at a safe and effective dosing regimen sometimes requires a substantial amount of time and patience. Most drugs need to be titrated gradually to reach

TABLE 18.2 COMMON DRUGS FOR THE TREATMENT OF NEUROPATHIC PAIN

Drug Category	Examples	Dosing	Common Side Effects	Monitoring
Tricyclic antidepressants (TCA)	Amitriptyline, nortriptyline, desipramine, imipramine (names end with *ine*)	Doses of the different TCAs are similar—usually between 25 and 75 mg/day for pain. Can be taken once a day at night	Drowsiness, dry mouth, difficulty urinating. Increased risk for falls in older adults	Electrocardiogram monitoring may be required when higher doses are prescribed, especially in people with heart conditions. Multiple drug interactions
Serotonin–norepinephrine reuptake inhibitors (SNRI)	Duloxetine (Cymbalta)	30–120 mg once a day	Dry mouth, tiredness, nausea.	Typically no special monitoring. Both drugs require dose reduction if kidney or liver function is impaired
	Venlafaxine (Effexor, others)	75–225 mg/day	Dry mouth, nervousness, drowsiness; increased blood pressure with higher doses	

Antiepileptics—gabapentin and pregabalin	Gabapentin (Neurontin, others)	Gabapentin—300–1200 mg 3 times a day (some formulations such as Horizant or Gralise are taken twice a day)	Dizziness, tiredness, weight gain, swelling of the feet and ankles	None typically. Pay attention to allergic reactions. Both drugs need dose adjustment if kidney function is impaired
	Pregabalin (Lyrica)	75–300 mg twice a day		
Antiepileptics—Carbamazepine and oxcarbazepine *Mainly useful in a neuropathic pain condition called trigeminal neuralgia, causing pain in the face*	Carbamazepine (Tegretol, others) Oxcarbazepine (Trileptal)	*Carbamazepine:* Usually 200–800 mg/day. Frequency depending on the brand *Oxcarbazepine:* usually 900–1800 mg/day	May cause serious skin rashes and white blood cell changes; may affect liver function	Periodic blood tests for liver function and blood chemistry required. Multiple drug–drug interactions!

(continued)

TABLE 18.2 CONTINUED

Drug Category	Examples	Dosing	Common Side Effects	Monitoring
Lidocaine patch *Mainly useful for localized neuropathic pain—e.g., pain after shingles (postherpetic neuralgia)*	Lidocaine 5% patch (e.g., Lidoderm)	Up to 3 patches at one time, apply for 12 hours, and then remove for 12 hours	Minimal side effects, mainly local skin irritation. Applying more than 3 patches may result in absorption of large amount of lidocaine to the blood, causing side effects	None
Capsaicin *Useful for localized neuropathic pain—e.g., pain after shingles (postherpetic neuralgia)*	Capsaicin is the active ingredient of chili peppers. Available as a cream or solution for skin application or as a prescription-only skin patch	Cream: (0.025–0.1% capsaicin, Zostrix, others) apply 3–4 times a day for 4–6 weeks to see a clinical effect Patch (8% capsaicin, Qutenza): Applied in the physician's office once every 3–6 months	Generally very safe. Causes burning sensation on the skin when applied. The 8% patch may cause substantial burning/painful sensation at the time of application and up to a few hours thereafter	Use gloves when applying, and wash hands with soap. Avoid contact with eyes and mouth because capsaicin causes a burning sensation!

the desired dose, and then within a couple of weeks you can typically determine whether the treatment works well for your pain. Given the numerous side effects and drug–drug interactions of many of these medications, consult your physician or the pharmacist every time you start a new prescription or OTC medication or discontinue using one.

Headaches

Headaches are among the most common type of chronic pain. Although many people use NSAID medications or acetaminophen (or their combination) for headaches, these drugs are often not sufficiently efficacious. In addition, using analgesics too frequently may cause a "medication overuse headache," when painkillers actually worsen the headache. One of the common types of chronic headache is migraine headache, and an accurate diagnosis can help choose the most appropriate treatment. Migraine headaches (often associated with nausea and increased sensitivity to noise and light) respond well to the *triptan* medications such as *sumatriptan* (Imitrex, others) and *rizatriptan* (Maxalt, others). Half a dozen different *triptans* exist, and your neurologist may help you find the most appropriate one for you. When the frequency of migraines is high (more than 3-4 attacks per month), you should discuss migraine prevention (prophylaxis) with your physician. Medications such as *propranolol* (a beta-blocker usually used for high blood pressure; see Chapter 11), *amitriptyline* (TCA discussed earlier in this chapter and in Chapter 17), *valproate* or *topiramate* (antiepileptic medications discussed in Chapter 16), taken on daily basis, or *erenumab* (Aimovig, injected once a month) can be helpful in reducing the frequency and the severity of migraine headaches. Many of these medications have substantial side effects, and your physician can help you find the safest and most efficacious treatment, based on your other conditions and medications you take.

Fibromyalgia and Other Functional Pain Syndromes

This group of chronic pain conditions has not been characterized very well. Collectively, they have been termed *functional pain syndromes or more recently, primary chronic pain syndromes,* and include conditions such as fibromyalgia, irritable bowel syndrome, and chronic pelvic pain. The exact mechanisms causing these pain syndromes are unclear (although research is ongoing), but they often coexist with other conditions such as depression, anxiety, fatigue, and insomnia. These pain syndromes are also more prevalent in women. Nondrug therapy, which includes physical, cognitive behavioral, and coping approaches, as discussed in the beginning of this chapter, is usually the one that provides long-term benefits, but there are also pharmacological options that can help. *Duloxetine* and *pregabalin* (described earlier for neuropathic pain) have been approved for fibromyalgia and can be used effectively in these conditions. *Milnacipran* (Savella) is another drug from the SNRI antidepressant category that has been approved for fibromyalgia. While opioid medications may provide some (mainly short-term) relief, the current evidence does not support their long-term use in these pain syndromes, and opioids are best avoided.

SPECIAL POPULATIONS

Older adults are often more sensitive to side effects of pain medications. Drugs generally should be started at lower doses and dose-titrated more slowly, with more frequent monitoring of side effects. Many of the drugs discussed in this chapter, including opioids, antidepressants, and antiepileptics, may cause drowsiness and increase the risk for falls. Older adults are also at a higher risk for stomach and intestinal bleeding from NSAIDs.

Pain management in *pregnancy* is a complex issue, but not impossible. None of the medications to treat pain are absolutely prohibited in pregnancy, but many have certain risks. Antiepileptics are probably the least safe. The risks of using antidepressants or opioids need to be carefully considered against the benefits from the treatment. Acetaminophen is considered the safest among analgesic medications. NSAIDs are considered safe in the second trimester (months 4 to 6 of pregnancy), but their use late in pregnancy may impose risks on formation of some of the heart structures of the developing fetus. In general, nonpharmacological approaches are preferred. At times, when the pain is localized, injection of local anesthetics and even steroids can be considered in consultancy with you treating physician. The important issue is that if you are planning pregnancy and have chronic pain problems, discuss the safest treatment strategy with your doctor before becoming pregnant.

IMPORTANT QUESTIONS TO ASK YOUR DOCTOR

- What realistic outcomes should I expect from the treatment (for each treatment)?
- What side effects should I expect from each of my analgesic drugs? What should I do if I experience these?
- Are there tests I need to schedule to monitor the safety of my drugs?
- What other drugs should I avoid in terms of drug interactions?

THINGS YOU CAN DO TO IMPROVE TREATMENT OUTCOMES

- Set realistic expectations from your pain management strategy and define your treatment objectives—what you want your treatment to achieve. A personal tip: complete pain relief may not be possible in chronic pain, at least not in one step. Step-by-step improvements may be more realistic to achieve.

- Keep a pain diary—in terms of both how severe your pain is and how much it interferes with your ability to be physically active, to work, and to interact with friends and family. For each new treatment, determine how much each of these parameters has changed. You can simply use a scale from 0 to 10, where **0** is no pain/interference and **10** is the worst pain/interference you can imagine. Discuss with your physician using simple but validated scales such as the Brief Pain Inventory for that purpose.

- Make yourself familiar with the effects of excessive doses of your drugs, particularly if you take opioids (in which case it is sleepiness, drowsiness, reduced breathing rate), and immediately consult with a doctor if you are concerned that your dose may be too high.

- Be as physically active as your pain allows. Ask a trained physical therapist to teach you exercises relevant to your pain and practice those daily at home.

- Try to learn strategies that distract your mind from pain (e.g., breathing, relaxation, mindfulness meditation, yoga). Practicing these on a regular basis can help a lot in the long run.

- Avoid drinking alcohol and using any substances that can cause drowsiness or impaired breathing.

VALUABLE RESOURCES FOR ADDITIONAL EDUCATION ON PAIN

I am not aware of a single, comprehensive, reliable source of pain education for patients. You probably realized from this chapter that chronic pain is not a single disease, and the various types of pain require different approaches and drugs and therefore a different focus on patient education. I am hoping this chapter provides enough details so that you can ask the right questions to achieve optimal pain management.

You can find some useful links and information here:

Pain Research Forum (PRF) website: http://www.painresearchforum.org/about/for-patients
Pain Toolkit website: https://www.paintoolkit.org/tools
Patient Resource page of the International Association for the Study of Pain (IASP): https://www.iasp-pain.org/Education/Content.aspx?ItemNumber=1723&navItemNumber=678

[19]

THYROID PROBLEMS

Restoring the Delicate Energetic Balance

The thyroid is a small, butterfly-shaped gland at the base of your neck. The thyroid gland produces thyroid hormones, T_3 (also called triiodothyronine) and T_4 (also called thyroxine), which control many activities in the body, primarily development of the central nervous system and metabolic processes related to energy expenditure.

Essentially, the thyroid gland produces and releases thyroid hormones as a response to a hormone called thyroid-stimulating hormone (TSH) which is produced by the pituitary gland in the brain. The release of TSH is triggered by the levels of thyroid hormones circulating in the blood. Low thyroid hormone levels in the blood prompt TSH release from pituitary to signal the thyroid gland to produce more thyroid hormones. Thyroid hormones affect almost every organ in the body and are involved in regulating a variety of processes, including metabolism, menstrual cycle, breathing, heart rate, and nervous system function. Both hormones, T_4 and T_3, have an *iodine* atom attached to them. Iodine is critical for thyroid hormone synthesis, but it is not very abundant in dietary sources; therefore, the occurrence of thyroid disorders varies based on the availability of iodine in the diet. If you look at the type of kitchen salt you use, you are likely to notice that the label reads "iodinized salt" (or iodized salt), especially if you live in the United States. Iodized salt is basically a regular salt, which is supplemented with very small amounts of iodine, to help prevent thyroid disorders associated with iodine deficiency.

A variety of thyroid disorders are known, from relatively harmless enlargement of the thyroid gland (goiter) to thyroid cancer. Women are much more likely than men to have thyroid problems: diseases associated with thyroid hormone secretion affect about 0.5% of men and 5% of women. This chapter will not focus on the pathology of thyroid disease but rather will briefly describe the most common conditions and refer to the drug treatment of two main consequences of thyroid disease: *hyperthyroidism,* resulting from too much thyroid hormone production; and *hypothyroidism,* resulting from insufficient production of thyroid hormones.

Hyperthyroidism can result from a variety of conditions such as Graves' disease (disease of the immune system that triggers too much production of thyroid hormone), inflammation of the thyroid gland, or development of benign or malignant nodules in the thyroid. The prevalence is somewhere between 0.5 and 2% (one of every 50 to 200 people). Hyperthyroidism may cause multiple symptoms, including nervousness, irritability, sleeping difficulties, hand tremors, irregular heartbeats, weight loss, diarrhea, and mood swings. However, different people with hyperthyroidism may have a different set of symptoms.

Hypothyroidism can result from *Hashimoto's disease* (another disease of the immune system that leads to damage of the thyroid tissue and **reduces** the production of thyroid hormones), from surgical removal of the thyroid gland, and from exposure to excessive amounts of iodine or to certain drugs. The symptoms of hypothyroidism vary but may include fatigue, weight gain, constipation, dry skin, decreased sweating, depression, and muscle, and joint pain.

TREATMENT GOALS

Treatment goals in hyperthyroidism or hypothyroidism usually include the following:

- Reverse the complaints and symptoms associated with hyperthyroidism or hypothyroidism
- Normalize TSH and thyroid hormone levels
- Prevent severe hyperthyroidism (*thyroid storm*) or severe hypothyroidism (*myxedema*)
- Improve emotional well-being and quality of life
- Support normal maintenance of pregnancy, if relevant
- Reduce nodule (goiter) size, if relevant
- Maintain normal bone density and prevent osteoporosis (in *hyper*thyroidism)

TREATMENT APPROACH

The treatment of thyroid disease is focused on replacing the lacking hormones in hypothyroidism, or decreasing thyroid hormone production in hyperthyroidism, and on controlling the appropriate symptoms. Several laboratory tests are available to assess thyroid *homeostasis* and function, most of these measuring the levels of TSH, as well as T_4 and T_3 hormones. If you suffer from some kind of thyroid disorder or have symptoms suggesting a thyroid disease, your doctor is likely to order one or more of these tests (or additional blood or imaging tests) both for determining your baseline thyroid function and for monitoring your treatment success.

SPECIFIC DRUGS

Hypothyroidism treatment is usually pharmacological and includes replacement of the thyroid hormones. Table 19.1 describes the common drugs used to replace thyroid hormones. The general approach of treating *hyperthyroidism* is somewhat different. There are three main modalities: surgical removal of the thyroid, treatment with radioactive iodine to chemically destroy cells in the thyroid gland, or antithyroid drugs such as *propylthiouracil* (PTU) and *methimazole* (Table 19.2). Generally, the long-term efficacy of all three approaches for hyperthyroidism is quite similar; therefore, the ultimate choice will depend on your preferences and coexisting conditions as well as the individual risks and benefits of each intervention. In addition to correcting the thyroid hormone imbalance, your doctor can offer symptomatic treatment of hyperthyroidism manifestations.

DRUG-RELATED SPECIAL ISSUES

The SAME-SAME-SAME program of the American College of Endocrinology/American Academy of Clinical Endocrinologists highlights the importance of consistent dosing (same medication, same dosage, same time) when treating thyroid disease because the balance is very delicate and even minor differences in absorption of various generic brands can cause a misbalance. The specific brand of thyroid medicine that you take is less important than the issue that once the desired T_3–T_4–TSH balance is achieved with a certain drug, or drug combination, stick to it.

Thyroid hormones (those for treating *hypo*thyroidism) usually need to be taken on an empty stomach with a full glass of water about 30 to 60 minutes before taking any food, vitamins, or medications. This is because some types of food, such as dairy products or

TABLE 19.1 COMMON DRUGS FOR TREATING HYPOTHYROIDISM

Drug	Doses	Administration Tips
L-thyroxine (synthetic T_4, also called levothyroxine) (Synthroid, Levoxyl, others)	Generally the treatment of choice in hypothyroidism. Usual starting doses 100–150 mcg/day in adults, 50–100 mcg/day in older adults. Once a day treatment	If you have heart disease or are more sensitive to metabolic effects of T_4, your initial dosages may be lower (e.g., 25 mcg) and dose increases more gradual. Best taken on empty stomach (30–60 minutes before breakfast), avoid taking with antacids
Liothyronine (synthetic T_3) (Cytomel)	Maintenance dose 25–75 mcg/day. Once a day	Recommended starting dose is 25 mcg/day. In some conditions, starting doses of 5 mcg are warranted
Liotrix (Thyrolar): a combination of *synthetic* T_3 and T_4 hormones	Available in different ratios (1:8 and 1:4) of T_3:T_4 per tablet	Usual initiation at low dose, with 50% increments in dose every 2–3 weeks, as necessary, based on free T_4/thyroid-stimulating hormone lab results and symptoms

(continued)

TABLE 19.1 CONTINUED

Drug	Doses	Administration Tips
Desiccated thyroid or thyroid extract (dry powder derived from a thyroid gland of pork or beef) *These are not FDA-approved drugs* and are available from various manufacturers as a dietary supplement	Initial: 30 mg orally once a day. Can be increased by 15 mg per every 2–3 weeks to achieve normal T_3 and T_4 levels in blood. Usual maintenance: 60–120 mg/day of the extract	Because this is an animal-derived product, there is a higher risk for variability in the active components from batch to batch. Contains a mixture of T_4 (approx. 80%) and T_3 (approx. 20%) hormones—which is different from the 90-to-10% ratio in humans

coffee, and some drugs can interfere with *levothyroxine* (T_4) absorption by either binding to it in the gut or changing stomach acidity and thus affecting the breakdown of levothyroxine tablets. However, if you have been taking your thyroid medication in a certain way, such as after breakfast, and your symptoms and lab tests are balanced, then continue with the same routine. Avoid changes. Remember: SAME-SAME-SAME!

Certain drugs can negatively interact with thyroid hormones and affect their absorption and thus effectiveness. Some examples follow:

- *Cholestyramine* and *colestipol* (resin binders for treating high cholesterol levels as discussed in Chapter 12). These drugs

TABLE 19.2 DRUGS FOR TREATING HYPERTHYROIDISM

Drug	Doses	Side Effects	Mode of Action and Administration Tips
Methimazole (Tapazole)	Usually initiated at 10–40 mg/day and maintained at 5–15 mg/day based on symptoms and blood test results. Dosage may be different for preparation for surgery or radioactive iodine therapy	Common side effects: nausea, skin rash. Rare side effects: toxicity to white or red blood cells, and liver toxicity. Generally side effects less common than with PTU (below)	The mechanism of action is not completely understood, but they inhibit the synthesis of T_4 hormone in the thyroid gland and the conversion of T_4 hormone to its more active T_3 form. It may take 2–8 weeks to observe symptomatic changes with PTU treatment
Propylthiouracil (PTU)	Usually initiated at 150–400 mg/day and maintained at 100–150 mg/day. The daily amount to be taken in 2–3 divided doses. In most cases PTU is second choice after methimazole	Common side effects: skin rash, bitter taste, may cause toxicity to white and red blood cells. Potentially can cause liver toxicity	

(continued)

TABLE 19.2 CONTINUED

Drug	Doses	Side Effects	Mode of Action and Administration Tips
Beta-blockers such as propranolol, atenolol, and metoprolol (see Chapter 11)	Doses vary depending on the drug and formulation—between once a day (atenolol) and 4 times a day (immediate-release propranolol)	Side effects: low blood pressure, decreased heart rate, headaches. Propranolol is less recommended if you have diabetes (see Chapter 14) or asthma (see Chapter 15)	Beta-blockers provide symptomatic relief only for manifestations such as increased heartbeats, nervousness, and hand tremors. Beta-blockers do not modify the release of T_3/T_4 from the thyroid gland
Calcium channel blocker—diltiazem (Cardizem, others; see Chapter 11)	Daily doses between 80 and 360 mg. The frequency of administration depends on formulation—typically two or three daily doses	Side effects: low blood pressure, decreased heart rate, sore throat, constipation	Symptomatic relief only, usually reserved for patients who cannot tolerate beta-blockers. Diltiazem interacts with many drugs!

reduce the absorption of thyroid hormones and should be taken 4 to 6 hours before, or 2 hours after, your thyroid hormones.

- Antacids containing aluminum or calcium, as well as iron supplements, can also substantially impair thyroid hormone absorption. Those should also be separated from thyroid hormones and avoided 4 to 6 hours before and 2 hours after thyroid medication intake.

Excessive doses of thyroid hormones may predispose individuals to bone loss, osteoporosis, and irregular heartbeats; therefore, periodic monitoring of symptoms as well as blood hormone levels is important. Short-term side effects of excessive thyroid hormone doses include the typical symptoms of hyperthyroidism such as nervousness, irritability, loose stools, weight loss, frequent heartbeats, and tremor.

Thyroid disorders can affect other drugs' status because they can affect the general metabolic rate in the body. Drugs such as *warfarin* (see Chapter 13), *insulin* (see Chapter 14), *theophylline* (see Chapter 15), *digoxin* (for certain heart rate abnormalities), and *corticosteroids* (for various inflammatory diseases) may require dose adjustments in patients with hypothyroidism or hyperthyroidism.

On the other hand, there are several drugs that may cause hypothyroidism. Among the important ones are *lithium* (used to treat bipolar disorder), *sertraline* (to treat depression; see Chapter 17), *amiodarone* (to treat certain heart rhythm problems; *amiodarone* can also cause *hyperthyroidism*), *sulfonylurea* drugs (to treat diabetes; see Chapter 14), *interferon-alpha* and *interleukin-2* (both used in cancer management).

Monitoring

Usually blood tests for thyroid function will be taken after a steady state has been achieved, roughly 2 to 3 months after you start treatment or change the dose of your thyroid medications. After reaching the goals, your doctor will typically re-evaluate thyroid hormone levels every 12 months (or more frequently if misbalance is suspected).

Adjunct Treatment for Hyperthyroidism

Sometimes drugs that do not directly affect thyroid function can help control hyperthyroidism *symptoms* such as increased heart rate, tremor, and nervousness. These include beta-blockers and the calcium channel blocker diltiazem described in Table 19.2. These are often used as "bridge therapy" before surgery or radiation, or while waiting for the full effect of *propylthiouracil (PTU)* or *methimazole* (usually 2 to 8 weeks).

Administration of high amounts of **iodine supplements** acutely suppresses thyroid hormone secretion. *Potassium perchlorate* and *potassium iodide* (Lugol's solution) have been historically used to treat hyperthyroidism but are not safe for long-term treatment. They are sometimes used today in special cases for short-term control of hyperthyroidism, such as around surgery.

In treatment-resistant situations, when *methimazole* or PTU fail to control your hyperthyroidism, your doctor may consider prescribing additional drugs that reduce the effects of thyroid hormones, such as *cholestyramine* or *lithium*.

SPECIAL POPULATIONS

Pregnancy

Hypothyroidism during pregnancy can have negative consequences, including premature birth and miscarriage. If the hypothyroidism results from insufficient iodine intake in the pregnant woman's diet, this can have further negative consequences because thyroid hormone production by the developing baby's thyroid gland is critical for proper development of its brain, and the only source of iodine for the baby is its mother's diet. Ensuring proper iodine intake during pregnancy and treating any existing hypothyroidism are therefore very important.

Hyperthyroidism in pregnancy, on the other hand, is another challenging issue. *Methimazole* and *PTU*, drugs usually used for treating hyperthyroidism, may both have adverse outcomes in pregnancy. Although *methimazole* generally has fewer side effects than *PTU*, it probably bears higher risk to the fetus if administered to the mother in the first trimester of pregnancy. *PTU* might be preferable between the two in pregnancy and breastfeeding for hyperthyroidism treatment. However, as new evidence becomes available, these recommendations might change.

If you have hyperthyroidism and are planning a pregnancy, sometimes a treatment with radioactive iodine 4 to 6 months before the planned pregnancy will be the best choice because it will eliminate the need for drug therapy during pregnancy. Once the thyroid gland is inactive (with surgery or radioactive iodine), you will be placed on thyroid hormone replacements, and when the T_4 and TSH balance (and symptom control) are achieved, conception can be attempted.

Thyroid hormones such as *levothyroxine* are safe in pregnancy. The key points are to plan ahead and to consult with your endocrinologist if you are planning pregnancy.

IMPORTANT QUESTIONS TO ASK YOUR DOCTOR

- What is causing my thyroid disease?
- What are the short-term and long-term goals of my treatment?
- Are there drugs and foods to avoid, considering my condition and treatment?
- Based on the brand of thyroid medication I am prescribed, what are the exact instructions for taking it?
- How frequently should I perform my thyroid function blood tests? How will I be notified if I need to change medication doses based on the test results?
- What are the signs that my thyroid drug is causing too little or too much of an effect?

THINGS YOU CAN DO TO IMPROVE TREATMENT OUTCOMES

- Stick to the "same drug, same dose, same time" principle with thyroid medications.
- Perform all scheduled blood tests for determining plasma T_4 and TSH levels to assess the effectiveness of your treatment.
- Talk to your doctor if your symptoms are not controlled. Although frequently the symptoms will reflect the lab test results, the treatment goal is to help you, not the lab tests. Lab norms exist for reference values, and you don't need

to be right in the middle of the norm range. Based on your symptoms (and other conditions), your doctor may decide on blood test goals aimed toward the lower or the higher end of thyroid hormone level norms.

- If you are planning pregnancy, consult your doctor at least 5 months before your planned conception.

VALUABLE RESOURCES FOR ADDITIONAL EDUCATION ON THYROID DISEASE

American Thyroid Association: http://www.thyroid.org/thyroid-information/

National Institutes of Health: https://www.niddk.nih.gov/health-information/endocrine-diseases/

[20]

INFECTIONS

Destroying the Invaders while Saving the Host

Infections cost about $120 billion dollars to the US economy and account for 138 million visits to a healthcare setting per year. Of these, about 22 million are visits to hospital emergency departments. These visits account for roughly 16% of all emergency hospital admissions, with leading causes being pneumonia (lung), skin, blood, and urinary tract infections.

Infection, or infectious disease, is defined as the invasion to the body and multiplication of microorganisms such as viruses, bacteria, or parasites. In most cases, the microorganisms are acquired from outside of the body. However, in some cases, bacteria that normally live in our body and are not infectious (e.g., *Escherichia coli* in the intestine) can get to the urinary tract or the bloodstream and cause serious infections. Most infections are accompanied by symptoms, but depending on whether the infection is localized to a certain organ (skin, eye, lungs) or spread through the blood to various organs, these symptoms may vary. Fever is among the most common indicators of an infection, but it won't accompany all infections. It is important to know, therefore, that an infection may be asymptomatic (without symptoms) in some cases, depending on the offending microorganism and the person's age, condition, and immune function. For example, pneumonia caused by certain types of bacteria such as *Streptococcus* species is likely to result in high temperature and substantial cough, with large production of mucus, while other types of bacteria, such as *Mycoplasma* species, may cause pneumonia that would be accompanied by low-grade (or absence of) fever, some dry cough, and tiredness. Your physician is trained to recognize and diagnose infections, but it is more challenging when the symptoms are less profoundly expressed. Another example of an asymptomatic infection would be when an individual contracts HIV; he or she may experience no symptoms until the infection becomes more severe.

Our immune system is equipped with sophisticated mechanisms to kill bacteria, viruses, and other microorganisms that invade our body. If we are infected with a small amount of bacteria, we may not have any symptoms of infection if the immune system effectively handles the threat. However, once the load of microorganisms reaches a critical mass, our body might not be able to get rid of it efficiently. Interestingly, this critical mass might be very different based on your age, immune system function, and additional diseases or medications that affect your immune system.

Infections are very diverse, and their severity and prognosis are always about the specific three-way interaction between (1) the microorganism (i.e., the pathogen), (2) the anatomical location of the infection in the body, and (3) the individual host (the person). It is beyond the scope of this book to cover the main types of infections, their epidemiology, and their treatment. The range of pathogens is also very large, from viruses (influenza, hepatitis) and retroviruses (e.g., HIV) to fungal infections and numerous bacterial infections. Since this book is about safe and effective drug therapy and we cannot possibly cover all aspects of infections, I will focus this chapter on drugs used to treat bacterial infections in the out-of-hospital setting (not covering viral and fungal infections, or in-hospital treatments of infections). Antibacterial medications are referred to as *antibiotics,* and this chapter will discuss their use in treating infections.

TREATMENT GOALS

The goals of the antibiotic treatment depend on the type of infection. In most infections, the goal is to get rid of the offending pathogen or to minimize its load to an extent that it can be cleared by the immune system. This, in turn, will alleviate your symptoms and also minimize the risk of people around you contracting the pathogen ("Why should I take my medications?" section in Chapter 5 can help refine these goals in each case).

The strongest weapon that bacteria have is their ability to divide and grow rapidly. The time that it takes a group of bacteria to double their number (termed *generation time*) varies, but if we consider a certain strain of *Streptococcus,* for example, it may only take about 1 hour. At a glance, you might think that this is not a huge growth rate. Let's assume a person was initially infected with *1000* bacteria. As you can see in Table 20.1, within 24 hours, this number can rise to more than *16 billion* bacteria!

This formula is not a constant but an approximation, and there are several factors that can determine this growth rate. One particularly important factor is the body temperature. Because temperature appears to be important for bacterial growth, some guidance on managing high body temperature (fever) is presented next.

Managing Fever

Most bacteria will grow more slowly at higher temperatures (e.g., 38.6° C [101.8° F]) than at lower temperatures (e.g., 36.6° C [98° F]). In fact, the difference in growth rate in these two temperatures can

TABLE 20.1 EXAMPLE OF BACTERIA GENERATION TIME

Generation Time	Number of Bacteria Present
0 (initial infection)	1000
1 hour	2000
2 hours	4000
3 hours	8000
12 hours	4,096,000
24 hours = 24 generation times	16,777,216,000

be more than two-fold! Therefore, fever, as the body's defense mechanism, can help slow down bacterial growth and help antibiotics work. Consequently, the recommendation typically is not to take fever-reducing (antipyretic) medications for low-grade fever, but rather to take them when your temperature is high, above 38.5° C (~102° F), to prevent discomfort and dehydration. It is possible that brain damage can occur at temperatures higher than 42° C (~107° F), but even untreated infections rarely produce that kind of fever.

Many pediatricians recommend not treating temperature below 38.3° C (101° F) in children. It makes a lot of sense, but remember that this recommendation *excludes* infants younger than 6 months, in whom any temperature of 38° C (100.5° F) or higher requires an immediate evaluation by a physician. In children, particularly those younger than 5 years, high temperature may increase the risk for febrile seizures (colloquially called *fever fit*). However, these febrile seizures (1) are usually harmless and (2) are not always related to temperature above a certain threshold.

TREATMENT APPROACH

The antibiotic treatment goal is to halt bacterial division and growth. Most antibiotics kill bacteria without killing host (human) cells, by taking advantage of certain characteristics of bacteria that human cells don't share. The two major mechanisms by which antibiotic drugs work are the following:

1. Bacteria are tiny cells that come in various sizes and shapes. Certain strains of bacteria have a cell wall (as opposed to a cell membrane in human cells) that consists of a structure called *peptidoglycan*. For these bacteria to divide and grow, they need to build a lot of cell walls because every new cell needs its wall. Many antibiotics, *penicillin* for example, work by inhibiting the synthesis of the bacterial cell wall. The result is that bacteria cannot create a new cell wall, and they die. At the same time, these antibiotics do not affect the division of human cells.

2. Bacteria also have DNA. To divide and grow, bacteria need to synthesize new DNA molecules, but some of the processes (and the involved proteins) are different from the ones in humans. Utilizing these differences, the second major mechanism of antibiotic action is to penetrate into the bacteria and interfere with various proteins that participate in the synthesis of DNA or other key molecules, and by doing so to prevent bacteria from dividing and growing.

When a person has (a suspected) bacterial infection, there are two general approaches to antibiotic treatment: *empiric* treatment and *definitive* treatment.

The *empiric* approach is based on your doctor's suspicion about which microorganism has caused the infection, without identifying the offending organism. If we know that 95% of people who present with a sore throat, fever, and certain findings on physician's examination will have an infection caused by the bacterium *Streptococcus,* then there might be no need to test for the presence of bacteria. Consequently, someone who presents with the previous symptoms should be treated with an antistreptococcal antibiotic drug. And if your physician also knows that in most cases these bacteria will not be resistant to a treatment with, for example, *penicillin,* then it makes a lot of sense to treat you *empirically* without the additional cost and time required to perform the tests to identify the offending bacteria and their sensitivity to antibiotics. Although the empiric approach carries a certain risk associated with not diagnosing the infection accurately, it is nevertheless a common and cost-effective approach for many infections in the outpatient setting.

In a different scenario, *empiric* treatment might not be the best approach. If you had a compromised immune function (e.g., with cancer) and have a severe blood infection, it will be critical to identify the offending microorganism as soon as possible. Moreover, since the resistance of bacteria to antibiotics grows globally, in serious cases there is a need to test to which antibiotics your bacteria are sensitive to, and treat accordingly. In these cases, the treatment will be usually divided into two stages:

1. Your physician will take an appropriate sample (e.g., blood or urine, depending on the infection) and send it to the lab for identification of the offending bacteria and then to test for antibiotic sensitivity in order to determine the definitive treatment.

2. After the sample has been obtained, an *empiric* treatment will be prescribed until the lab results come back. This empiric treatment will usually include broad-range antibiotic therapy

with a single drug or a combination of drugs. Broad-range antibiotics kill a wide range of different bacteria. When the lab results come back, demonstrating to which antibiotic(s) the offending bacteria are sensitive, you will be switched to *definitive* treatment if the initial antibiotic choice was inappropriate.

In the case of communicable infections (i.e., those that can be spread to another person), it is important to remember that the goals are not only to treat your infection but also to prevent others from being infected. It is, therefore, important to ask your doctor about the ways your infection may spread and the appropriate approaches to prevent that spread.

One of the main reasons that antibiotic treatments fail is the lack of patient adherence to the prescribed treatment. On average, between one and two of every five people who are prescribed an antibiotic do not adhere to the treatment properly. This most often includes missing doses or not completing the full prescribed sequence. There is plenty of research demonstrating that lack of adherence results in higher risk for treatment failure and complications of the infection. Therefore, it is of critical importance that you follow the physician orders regarding your daily regimen and the duration of antibiotic treatment. If you experience side effects or are considering stopping the treatment for any other reason, discuss it with your physician first.

SPECIFIC DRUGS

A huge amount of antibiotic medications exist. For brevity, and because the patient responsibility is primarily relevant when taking medications at home, I will focus here on those administered orally and not those given by injection in a hospital setting. The main groups of antibiotics are presented in Table 20.2, which describes

TABLE 20.2 COMMON GROUPS OF ORALLY ADMINISTERED ANTIBIOTICS

Drug Class	Common Examples	Site of Action	Most commonly Used to Treat which Infections?	Administration Tips and Precautions
Penicillins	Penicillin V/VK, amoxicillin, amoxicillin with clavulanic acid (Augmentin)	Bacterial wall	Ear and throat infections, sinusitis, respiratory tract infections	Most penicillins such as penicillin V are better absorbed on an empty stomach, but this is not a critical issue. Amoxicillin/clavulanic acid combination should be taken with or after a meal to prevent upset stomach
Cephalosporins	Cephalexin (Keflex), cefuroxime (Ceftin)	Bacterial wall	Respiratory infections, skin infections, urinary tract infections	Cefuroxime should be taken after a meal, which increases its bioavailability. For other cephalosporins, food intake does not affect absorption significantly

| Macrolides | Erythromycin (Eryc, EES), azithromycin (Zithromax), clarithromycin (Biaxin) | Inside the bacterial cell | Respiratory infections, acne, ear and throat infections, genital infections | The absorption of erythromycin is improved on an empty stomach; however, it may frequently cause upset stomach and should be taken with food to prevent that. Macrolide antibiotics (especially erythromycin) potentially interact with many drugs because they are inhibitors of CYP enzymes in the liver. They may also cause certain changes in heart rhythm, especially with other drugs that act on heart conductivity. Check with your doctor or pharmacist |

(*continued*)

TABLE 20.2 CONTINUED

Drug Class	Common Examples	Site of Action	Most commonly Used to Treat which Infections?	Administration Tips and Precautions
Fluoroquinolones	Ciprofloxacin (Cipro), ofloxacin (Floxin), levofloxacin (Levaquin)	Inside the bacterial cell	Urinary tract infections, prostate inflammation, gastrointestinal infections	Fluoroquinolones are better absorbed on an empty stomach. If you take iron for treating anemia, avoid taking it 2 hours before or after fluoroquinolones because iron may decrease their absorption and efficacy. May cause heart conduction abnormalities in high-risk patients, similarly to macrolides. Traditionally, quinolone use in *children* and *pregnant women* has been avoided, owing to adverse outcomes based on animal research. Recent studies indicate that fluoroquinolones might be safer in these patients than previously thought

		Inside the bacterial cell	Urinary tract infections, prophylaxis of certain lung infections in immune-compromised people	There might be an increased risk for certain blood abnormality (called *hemolytic anemia*) in patients with the lack of G6PD enzyme. Consult your doctor if you are G6PD deficient. It may cause increased sensitivity of skin to sunlight; wear sunscreen
Co-trimoxazole	Sulfamethoxazole/ trimethoprim (Bactrim)			
Lincosamide antibiotics	Clindamycin (Cleocin, Dalacin)	Inside the bacterial cell	Gingival and periodontal infections, skin infections, abdominal infections, treatment of abscesses	Take with a full glass of water. If you experience severe watery/ bloody diarrhea, stop the treatment and immediately contact your doctor *Vaginal suppositories are available*. Verify correct method of administration

(*continued*)

TABLE 20.2 CONTINUED

Drug Class	Common Examples	Site of Action	Most commonly Used to Treat which Infections?	Administration Tips and Precautions
Tetracyclines	Tetracycline, minocycline (Minocin), doxycycline (Adoxa, Doryx)	Inside the bacterial cell	Mainly acne. Also used for treating genital infections, Lyme disease, and certain rare infections	Take with a full glass of water. Tetracycline is to be taken on empty stomach; especially avoid dairy products 2 hours before and 1 hour after taking tetracycline because food will reduce the drug's absorption. The absorption of minocycline and doxycycline is less affected by food or dairy products. The use of tetracyclines beyond the first trimester of pregnancy and in children younger than 8 years is generally not recommended because of potential problems with teeth and bones

| Nitroimidazoles | Metronidazole | Inside the bacterial cell | Respiratory infections, genital infections, abdominal infections | Metronidazole should be taken with food to decrease gastrointestinal upset. Avoid alcohol during metronidazole treatment and for 2–3 days after stopping it. Metronidazole should be avoided in pregnancy, especially in the first trimester. *Vaginal suppositories are available.* Verify the correct route of administration |

G6PD = glucose-6-phosphate dehydrogenase.

a few examples for each group of antibiotic drugs along with a few precautions and administration details.

DRUG-RELATED SPECIAL ISSUES

If Table 20.2 described a medication that you were prescribed (or that is otherwise somehow relevant to you), you will find in the following sections a bit more detailed description on the undesired effects of the drug, which should help you use it in a safer manner.

Penicillins (e.g., *Penicillin VK, Amoxicillin*)

Penicillin allergy is the most common medication allergy, reported to occur in up to 5 to 10% of people. Although the true prevalence is probably lower (and many of the penicillin allergy cases are not true allergies but rather cases of side effects such as rash), serious anaphylactic infections do occur with penicillin. If you have developed a serious allergic reaction to one type of penicillin, it is best to avoid all penicillins. Otherwise, penicillins are generally safe medications and can also be prescribed to pregnant women and very young children. Concerns about toxicity to the kidneys exist when administered at high doses in combination with other drugs that can harm the kidneys, especially in individuals who already have preexisting kidney problems.

Cephalosporins (e.g., *Cephalexin, Cefuroxime*)

Cephalosporins are structurally similar to penicillin antibiotics. About 10% of people who are allergic to penicillin may also have an allergy to cephalosporins. Usually, an allergy to penicillin is not a reason to avoid cephalosporins completely, but if someone had a serious anaphylactic reaction to penicillin, and alternative therapies are available, it is reasonable to choose the alternative. Cephalosporins are generally considered safe, but they also possess a small risk for kidney toxicity similarly to penicillins, again depending on the dose, other medications, and preexisting kidney disease.

Macrolides (e.g., *Erythromycin, Clarithromycin, Azithromycin*)

Macrolides (drugs ending with *mycin*) are generally quite safe, but there are two key points to be aware of when taking macrolides for treating an infection. The first point, as I briefly mentioned in Table 20.2, is that some macrolides (e.g., *erythromycin* and *clarithromycin*) are inhibitors of cytochrome P-450 (CYP) enzymes (see Chapters 3 and 8) and may seriously interact with other drugs. Their effect on CYP inhibition will result in increased blood concentrations (and potential toxicity) of the other, affected drug. Such serious interactions are likely with *statin* drugs (e.g., *simvastatin*), some hypertension drugs (e.g., *felodipine* and *amlodipine*), and many other medications. The second point is that macrolides may cause a certain pattern of changes in heart rhythm (called QT interval prolongation), which is detectable on electrocardiogram (ECG). Many psychiatric drugs, antifungal drugs, and other antibiotics such as *co-trimoxazole* or *fluoroquinolones* (discussed later), when combined with macrolides, further increase the risk for such heart rhythm abnormalities. If you are prescribed a macrolide on top of your other medications, it is worth double-checking with your doctor or pharmacist if the macrolide is safe for you. The most common side effect associated with macrolide antibiotics is upset stomach.

Fluoroquinolones (e.g., *Ciprofloxacin, Ofloxacin, Moxifloxacin*)

Fluoroquinolones (drugs ending with *floxacin*) can increase the sensitivity of the skin to sunlight. If you are 60 years or older, or receiving steroid treatment, or have received an organ transplant, these drugs can also increase the risk for inflammation and damage to tendons (e.g., the Achilles tendon). *Fluoroquinolones* are typically avoided in children younger than 8 years for similar reasons. As with macrolides, you should pay attention to the use of other drugs that may cause changes in the heart rhythm (e.g., certain antifungal and psychiatric drugs) *because the combination may increase the risk for arrhythmias.* Combining *fluoroquinolones* with *warfarin* (see Chapter 13) may increase the risk for bleeding.

Tetracyclines (e.g., *Minocycline, Doxycycline*)

Tetracyclines (end with *cycline*) increase the risk for sensitivity of the skin to sunlight; it is recommended to use sunscreen and avoid long exposure to sun if you are treated with a tetracycline. Inflammation of the esophagus (food pipe) has been reported with tablet dosage forms of *tetracyclines*, probably because of prolonged direct physical contact with the food pipe. Therefore, you should swallow *tetracyclines* with a full glass of water and not lie down for about 30 minutes afterward. Gastrointestinal symptoms such as cramps, diarrhea, and vomiting are the most frequently reported side effects of *tetracyclines*.

Co-trimoxazole (*Sulfamethoxazole/ Trimethoprim* Combination)

Sulfamethoxazole/trimethoprim (Bactrim, Sulfatrim) should be avoided if you are sensitive to sulfa drugs (sulfonamides). If you develop a rash while taking the drug, stop taking it and contact your provider. Individuals with a compromised immune system, particularly people with HIV/AIDS, who receive *co-trimoxazole* treatment are more likely to experience side effects such as rash than nonimmunocompromised individuals.

Metronidazole

If you take *metronidazole* (Metrogel, Flagyl), you should pay attention to any numbness or tingling that might develop in your feet and hands because this drug may (rarely) cause *neuropathy*, which is damage to the small nerve fibers that innervate the skin. There is also a rare risk for side effects in the central nervous system; if dizziness, visual disturbances, or problems with coordination or speech develop, stop the treatment and consult your doctor as soon as possible. *Metronidazole* can also cause skin rash and cause an unusual taste in the mouth. Avoid drinking alcohol during and a few days after *metronidazole* treatment because a severe reaction may occur from combining *metronidazole* with alcohol.

IMPORTANT QUESTIONS TO ASK YOUR DOCTOR

- Do I need definitive antibiotic treatment (or is empiric treatment sufficient)?
- Is my infection communicable? If yes, how does it spread, and what should I do to avoid infecting others?
- Do I have conditions that the prescribed antibiotic may adversely affect?
- Does the antibiotic negatively interact with any of my current drugs?

- How many times a day do I need to take my antibiotic, and how many days or weeks of treatment do I need to complete?
- Do certain types of food (e.g., dairy products) affect my antibiotic medication?
- How should I take it with regard to food?

THINGS YOU CAN DO TO IMPROVE TREATMENT OUTCOMES

- Follow your physician's orders. Some drugs have time-dependent killing of bacteria, which means you will need a certain amount of antibiotic to be present in your body for the treatment to succeed. Try your best not to miss antibiotic doses because missed doses can affect the success of your treatment.
- Learn about your infection and prevent spread if your infection is communicable. This may include frequent washing of hands, covering your cough, and not sharing tableware. For genital infections, it may include avoiding sexual contact with a partner and making sure to inform your partner about your infection, in case your partner also may require treatment.
- If you receive other prescription or over-the-counter drugs, make sure you have asked your doctor or the pharmacist about potential drug interactions.
- If you have a liver or kidney disease, make sure you have asked whether your antibiotic requires dosage adjustment, especially if the antibiotic prescriber is not your primary care doctor who knows you and your medical conditions.

VALUABLE RESOURCES FOR ADDITIONAL EDUCATION ON ANTIBIOTICS (AND MAINLY PREVENTION OF ANTIBIOTIC RESISTANCE)

Centers for Disease Control and Prevention: https://www.cdc.gov/getsmart/community/index.html

[21]

SUMMARY

The book has now guided you through the main principles of drug action. I have reviewed concepts such as pharmacodynamics, pharmacokinetics, side effects, and drug interactions. This book of course has not covered all aspects of drug therapy, but you should now have gained enough information to identify potential pitfalls regarding your drugs and to ask important questions in order to maximize the effectiveness and the safety of your treatment at home. I hope that Part II has provided some useful examples on the type of knowledge you should gain about each of your conditions and has given you tips that can help improve the outcomes of your therapy. The key components for successful drug therapy that were described in Chapter 5 involve answering the following three questions: **(1) WHY should I take my medications? (2) HOW should I take my medications? and (3) WHAT should I measure to track the treatment success?**

After you understand the goals of your treatment, what the ideal outcomes are, and what it is that each drug (or combination of drugs) tries to achieve, then make sure that you are well informed about the parameters to determine treatment success. This will help you achieve your goals. Creating a detailed table (see Table 21.1 as an example) in which you summarize your drugs, not just as a list but with

TABLE 21.1 EXAMPLE SUMMARY OF MEDICATION INSTRUCTIONS, GOALS, AND MONITORING

Drug	Dosing	Prescribed by	For Treating	Treatment Goal(s)	Blood Tests to Monitor	Extra Considerations
Amlodipine	10 mg once a day (9 a.m.)	Dr. H. Blood	High blood pressure	Blood pressure below 130/85 mm Hg	None	Avoid grapefruit juice. Monitor ankle swelling
Metformin	850 mg twice a day (after breakfast and dinner)	Dr. N. Zuckerman	Diabetes	*HbA$_{1c}$:* below 7% *Fingerstick glucose test:* **Before meals:** 80–130 mg/dL **After meals:** below 180 mg/dL	Glucose fingerstick (daily), HbA$_{1c}$ (every 3–6 months)	Examine feet daily for cuts/bruises. Eye exam once a year. Avoid NSAID medications if possible

HbA$_{1c}$ = hemoglobin A$_{1c}$, a measure of average blood glucose levels over the past 2–3 months; NSAID = nonsteroidal anti-inflammatory drug.

useful details about treatment monitoring and the drugs' main side effects, can substantially help you improve your treatment success.

An important component I tried to emphasize throughout the book is your role and responsibility as a patient in making sure that you are healthy and take your medications safely. Several health-care providers may be involved in your care, each having a unique understanding of certain components of your health. The opinions expressed in this book are in no way a substitute to recommendations from a healthcare provider who knows you; neither are they an individual medical advise. Rather, the familiarity with the key safety principles discussed throughout the book, can help you avoid some of the preventable side effects by asking the right questions.

Beyond the WHY, HOW, and WHAT questions that are critical to answer for the treatment of each of your conditions, you should also inquire about the drug-specific information on every new drug that you are prescribed. Answering the following set of core question can help you get the key information about your medications and make sure you take them appropriately.

1. What are the exact instructions for taking the drug (dose, frequency, time of day, relation to meals)?
2. How important is it to adhere to the medication? What if I miss a dose?
3. How long do I need to take this medication?
4. Are there certain foods or drinks I should avoid with this medication?
5. Am I taking any drugs that can increase the toxicity of the newly prescribed drug or that can be negatively affected by it?
6. Do I have conditions that the prescribed drug may adversely affect?

7. What side effects should I expect, and what are the warning signs of these side effects? Is this a drug with low therapeutic index?
8. Do I need periodic tests for monitoring the effectiveness or the safety of the drug? If yes, what are they, and how frequently should they be scheduled?
9. What other drugs should I avoid to prevent drug interactions?
10. Are the drug dose and frequency appropriate to my kidney and liver function (if there are problems with either)?

Tens of thousands of people die every year because of drug-related issues such as side effects and overdose, and this is in the United States alone. At least 50% of these cases are preventable, and my hope is that the information in this book will help you stay safe and healthy, away from these unfortunate statistics.

INDEX

Tables and figures are indicated by *t* and *f* following the page number.

For the benefit of digital users, indexed terms that span two pages (e.g., 52–53) may, on occasion, appear on only one of those pages.

rosuvastatin, 205
route of administration, 73

SABA. *See* short-acting beta-2 agonist
safety issues
    antidepressants, 301–2
    drug development process, 17
    hypertension medications, 194–95
    labeling, 144–45
    over-the-counter medications, 144
    See also prescription drug safety
St. John's wort, 155t
salicylic acid, 7, 154
salt
    and hypertension, 197
    iodized, 335–36
same-direction interactions, 134–35
SAME-SAME-SAME program, 338
seizures
    antihistamines and, 147–48
    epilepsy and, 267–71, 269t
selective serotonin reuptake inhibitors
    (SSRIs), 147, 229, 292–93, 294–99,
    295t, 300, 325
senna, 321
serotonin, 52, 292, 293f
serotonin–norepinephrine reuptake
    inhibitors (SNRIs), 294, 295t,
    300, 325, 326t
serotonin syndrome, 301–2
serotonin transporter, 292
sertraline, 295t, 302
Sertürner, Friedrich, 6–7
SGLT2 inhibitors. *See* sodium glucose
    cotransporter 2 inhibitors
shingles, 324
short-acting beta-2 agonist (SABA), 260–61
side effects
    ACE inhibitors, 188
    alcohol and, 139
    anticholinergic, 94–95
    beta-blockers, 191–92

and clinical trials, 22
complementary and alternative
    medicine, 155t
dealing with, 92–96
dose/concentration factors in, 88
gastrointestinal, 111, 309
individual variability in, 96–105
isotretinoin, 100–1
itching/rash, 90
metformin, 242
NSAIDs, 147
opioid analgesics, 101–5
orlistat, 150
over-the-counter medications, 145
and safety, 21–25
statin drugs, 205
warfarin, 99–100
signal transduction, 50
simvastatin, 117t, 205, 209–10, 363
sitagliptin, 239t, 243
sleep
    and depression, 289
    and respiratory function, 101–2
small intestine, 33
smoking
    and antidepressants, 306
    and antipsychotic drugs, 137–38
    and drug–drug interactions, 137–38
    and heart attack, 217
    and liver enzymes, 137
    removing enzyme-inducing effect
        of, 138
    risks associated with, 162
SNRIs. *See* serotonin–norepinephrine
    reuptake inhibitors
sodium glucose cotransporter 2
    (SGLT2) inhibitors, 244
spinal cord injury, 324
spirometry, 249–50
spironolactone, 193
SSRIs. *See* selective serotonin reuptake
    inhibitors